MOSBY'S
SPORTS THERAPY
TAPING
GUIDE

T0383235

MOSBY'S
SPORTS THERAPY
TAPING
GUIDE

ROBERT KENNEDY

Owner, Sports-Medics;
President, Fitness Tech Products Inc.,
Ottawa, Ontario
Canada

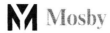

St. Louis Baltimore Boston Carlsbad Chicago Naples New York Philadelphia Portland
London Madrid Mexico City Singapore Sydney Tokyo Toronto Wiesbaden

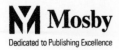

Mosby

Dedicated to Publishing Excellence

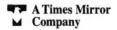

A Times Mirror Company

Printed in the United States of America

Transferred to Digital Printing 2008

PREFACE

This taping manual is geared to teach the novice taper while, at the same time it offers selected review points for the experienced person. This manual contains simple terminology to reach a broad base of individuals who are willing to learn or just review the many support techniques offered.

With this manual I hope to facilitate the learning process via clear, concise diagrams along with descriptive taping sequences. Using the knowledge and experience I have gained at University, National, International and Professional levels of athletic competition and the invaluable insight contributed by colleagues, I hope to stimulate some new thoughts to further the advancement of taping techniques. It is understood that there are many different techniques that exist, I have chosen those that are easy to learn and are very effective.

ACKNOWLEDGMENTS

I would like to thank the following individuals for their assistance in the development of this edition:

- David Berry (Certified Athletic Therapist) for his ideas and professional input

- Donna Koussaya (Certified Athletic Therapist) for her ideas and professional input

- Charlen Berry (Certified Athletic Therapist) and the Physabek Center for professional input

- Maxime Webb, for her expertise as copy editor

In addition, I would like to thank all friends and family for their support and encouragement.

TABLE OF CONTENTS

Mosby Sports Therapy Taping Guide

CHAPTER ONE

CHAPTER TWO

CHAPTER THREE

CHAPTER FOUR

THE PURPOSE OF TAPING

Before applying tape or elastic wraps, it is important to establish the purpose of the support techique. If the goal of using an elastic wrap is to decrease swelling, the wrap must start below or distal to the injury and work upwards or proximal toward the heart to force the swelling back into the circulatory system. Using elastic tape to secure a sterile dressing would mean that circulation would be compromised. If the aim of a support technique is to prevent a joint from entering a painful range, one must perform simple movement tests before the application of the tape.

When the tape job is complete, one must re-evaluate the movement to determine if the joint is moving in its painfree range. Too often inexperienced tapers simply read and follow the directions without any thought to what they are trying to accomplish. In addition, beginners forget to make sure that an athlete can function properly in his or her sport with a support technique in place. For example, the use of " buddy taping " does not work in a baseball glove. When applying tape and elastic wraps, always keep the purpose of the support technique in mind without losing sight of the athlete's sport and position.

PRINCIPLES OF ELASTIC WRAP

1- The purpose of an elastic wrap (tensor bandage) when used alone, is for compression or mild support.

2- When used with padding, support and compression are increased significantly.

3- Always apply the bandage from distal to proximal.

4- Always center the injury in the middle of the wrap.

5- Never allow the athlete to wear the bandage overnight.

6- Always check circulation after application.

7- Educate your athlete in the proper application at home.

8- For sports competitions, always secure the elastic wrap with elastic tape. Clips are not sufficient.

9- Never end the bandage on the inside (medial thigh, arm or ankle).

10- Wash the bandages frequently and between athletes.

MAIN FUNCTIONS OF TAPING & WRAPPING

1. To Provide Immediate First-Aid-

Elastic wraps, compression pads and open tape jobs work well in acute injury situations by decreasing swelling and eventually pain. Elastic tapes and wraps are used to provide compression and to hold dressings in place. Tape is also very beneficial during the rehabilitation process in that it provides protection but does not completely immobilize the joint. In combination with a proper rehabilitation program given by appropriate medical personnel, tape can facilitate the ultimate return to play for an athlete.

2. Taping To Prevent An Injury-

Preventative taping works well by decreasing the chance or limiting the extent of an injury, especially when combined with proper strength and balance programs. Prior to the use of such programs, one must consult the appropriate medical personnel. For certain injuries some strength exercises can actually do more harm than good.

Protective taping provides protection to the healing structures of an athlete who has suffered an injury. Although some injuries can improve with time, ligaments may take many weeks or months to completely heal. Protective taping can assist this long healing process while allowing the athlete to participate earlier in his or her sport.

For athletes who have a history of significant ligamentous injury producing joint laxity, preventative taping can be very useful. This is especially true for athletes competing in high risk sports (football, hockey, basketball... etc).

In all cases, whichever support technique has been applied, it is important that the athlete be able to function properly and adequately protect him/ herself during sport activity.

3. When Not To Apply Tape-

Although support techniques work well in some situations, they are not appropriate in others. Taping over any undiagnosed injury in order to allow an athlete to participate, could result in further injury. For example, a " running back " with a bad ankle injury may not be able to get out of the way of a hit and as a result could sustain a serious head, spinal or ligamentous injury. If there is ever any question that an injury exists be sure to have it professionally evaluated and rehabilitated. Never let an athlete return to play without written consent from their doctor. Tape should not be applied over broken or irritated skin. Athletes should always be asked if they have any allergies.

PRINCIPLES OF TAPE APPLICATION

1- The comfort of the person performing the taping procedure is crucial. The taping table height should be such that no bending at the waist is required.

2- When applying tape, follow the contours of the limb involved. Provide constant tension on the roll of tape to help eliminate wrinkles.

3- Have the athlete maintain the area to be taped in a pain free yet functional range or position (i.e., " The concept of grasping a ball " for a thumb tape job).

4- When taping over a muscle or tendon be sure to have the athlete contract the muscle involved.

5- When applying tape, overlap strips by at least one half the width of the tape to elliminate pinching or blisters.

6- Be careful not to cut off circulation with tape strips. Communicate with the athlete during the tape procedure and loosen strips as necessary. Tape should never be applied in a continuous manner.

7- To tear the tape, pinch each end with thumb and index finger while applying an outwards force. Tear the tape apart, do not twist it! A quick jerk of the tape will rip the ends more evenly.

4

8- Have the athlete check the function of the support technique once finished. If supported properly the limb will not enter a pain zone (painful range of motion). The direction of pull of the tape should be the opposite direction of the movement that causes pain.

SKIN PREPARATION

The skin should be shaved, washed and dried prior to tape application. All minor cuts and blisters should be cleaned, covered with ointment and/or " Spenco Second Skin " and a band-aid. When taping over nail beds, the use of a small band-aid can be helpful in preventing trauma to the structure. All sensitive areas of friction such as the achilles tendon, should be covered with a heel & lace pad and skin lubricant. If a heel and lace pad is not available a small gauze pad works well.

The area that is being taped should be sprayed lightly with tuf-skin adhesive spray. This will help the supported technique stay on longer. Underwrap is used to protect the skin from the irritation of the tape.

This is especially true for twice-a-day practices or when there are minor skin abrasions or allergies to the skin. When using underwrap in conjunction with taping spray, there is no need to shave the skin. Expect to lose some support.

TAPE REMOVAL

1- Tape should be removed immediately after its use as bacteria can build up

2- Be sure to use bandage scissors or tape cutters so that the skin does not become injured. Dip the end of the scissors or cutters in skin lubricant to facilitate the glide on the skin during the removal process. Follow the body's natural contours when removing the tape.

3- When pulling tape off of skin avoid tearing or irritating the skin. Pull the skin from the tape. Remove tape in a parallel motion to the skin surface rather than tearing tape up off the skin which can cause pain and even injury.

4- If using chemical removing agents to dissolve the tuf-skin spray, be sure to carefully wash the skin with soap and water afterwards.

5- Always watch for signs of skin breakdown such as dryness, redness or infection. These signs could be allergic reactions to the tape and/or the tuf-skin spray or remover. If allergic reactions occur, stop using the items immediately. Protect the whole area with underwrap to make sure that the tape does not contact the skin. Refer the athlete to the medical doctor for bad reactions should they occur. Athletes who cannot use tape or tuf-skin spray should consider prophylactic bracing.

6- After the tape has been removed, have the athlete apply a skin moisturizer to the area that was taped. This will help to replace lost moisture and prevent skin breakdown.

7- For the athlete with known allergies to tuf-skin spray, a hypo allergenic spray such as " skin prep " should be substituted. If the allergy is to the tape, then perhaps another brand of tape might be helpful. Adhesive backing will vary in chemical make- up from tape to tape.

TAPING REHABILITATION GUIDELINES

When tape is used on a regular basis for prevention of injury, it is recommended that the athlete maintain balance and strength for the involved joint.
Using the ankle joint as an example, balance work could be done by standing on one leg and then executing an arabesque gymnastics move (also known as a " 747 " stand by some therapists). Other techniques for improving balance could be conducted while using a wobble board or a " pro fitter ". These devices are found in many sports rehabilitation clinics.

Ankle strength work can be done by doing calf raises and by using rubber tubing to strengthen the muscles surrounding the ankle. Moving the ankle against the tubing into the position of eversion is helpful for lateral ankle sprains.

Ask your therapist or doctor for advice before doing any strengthening to a previously injured joint of any kind.

SPORTS THERAPIST TEAM KIT

BASIC CONTENTS

TUF-SKIN SPRAY
UNDERWRAP
WHITE ADHESIVE TAPE
ELASTIC TAPE (ELASTOPLAST)
ALCOHOL PREP PADS
TAPE REMOVER
STERI-STRIPS
SMALL COOLER
ROLLER GAUZE
ICE BAGS
SECOND SKIN
HEEL & LACE PADS
MOLESKIN
J-CLOTH
BACITRACIN
SKIN LUBRICANT, HAND LOTION
PROVIODINE (ANTISEPTIC SOLUTION)
BANDAGE SCISSORS
TONGUE DEPRESSORS
MIRROR, NAIL CLIPPERS
TOWELS, SCREWDRIVERS
PEN LIGHT, LATEX GLOVES
Q-TIPS
ASSORTED STERILE GAUZE PADS
KNIFE WITH RETRACTABLE BLADE
EMERGENCY ACTION PLAN & INFO.
PENS & PAPER
ATHLETE MEDICAL INFO CARD
TENSORS (VARIOUS SIZES)
TRIANGULAR BANDAGES
BUTTERFLY BANDAGES

OPTIONAL ITEMS

BLISTEX
DESENEX
EPSOM SALTS
LOZENGES
BULK COTTON
SALINE
SPACE BLANKET
EYE PATCHES
MAXI PADS
SUN SCREEN
TWEEZERS
ZINC OXIDE CREAM
CONTACT LENS KIT
SAFETY PINS
FELT

*** QUANTITIES WILL BE DETERMINED BY NUMBER OF
ATHLETES ON THE TEAM ***

8

SPORTS THERAPIST (PERSONAL ITEMS)

FANNY PACK CONTENTS
(EMERGENCY USE)

LATEX GLOVES (4 PAIR)
4 X 4 STERILE GAUZE (6)
3 X 3 STERILE GAUZE (6)
2 X 2 STERILE GAUZE (6)
TRIANGULAR BANDAGE (2)
SPACE BLANKET (1)
PEN LIGHT (1)
6" TENSOR (1)
4" TENSOR (1)
KNUCKLE BANDAGES (10)
ALCOHOL PREP PADS (10)
1/ 2" WHITE ADHESIVE TAPE (2 ROLL)
C.P.R. MOUTH SHIELD (1), POCKET MASK
Q-TIPS (10)

BELT HOLSTER

UNIVERSAL SCISSORS (1 PAIR)
UNIVERSAL SCREWDRIVER
RETRACTABLE CUTTING BLADE
BANDAGE SCISSORS

CHAPTER ONE

ANKLE TAPE-CLOSED GIBNEY BASKETWEAVE

ANKLE TAPE-CLOSED GIBNEY (OPTION)

COTTON-ANKLE WRAP (LOUISIANA)

ANKLE TAPE-OPEN GIBNEY

ACUTE ANKLE WRAP

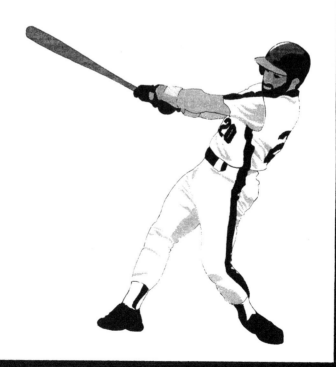

ANKLE TAPE-CLOSED GIBNEY BASKETWEAVE

PURPOSE: - To prevent inversion ankle sprains.

SUPPLIES: - tuf-skin spray
- underwrap
- skin lubricant

- 1 1/2" white adhesive tape
- heel & lace pads

IMPORTANT TEACHING POINTS:
SKIN PREPARATION
AND
BODY POSITIONING - The athlete's foot should be maintained in full
dorsiflexion (toes pointing upwards at all times.
Spray the front and back of the ankle with tuf-skin.
- Place a lubricated heel & lace pad on the front and one
on the back of the ankle (See Diagram A).
- Apply underwrap to the skin above the lateral and
medial malleolus, then apply underwrap to the
mid-forefoot using a " figure 8 ."

ANCHORS - Using 1 1/2" white adhesive tape, apply one anchor to
the mid-arch, it should cover the base of the 5th
metatarsal. Spread the toes apart with your fist before
securing the strip. Do not apply too much tension.
- Apply three overlapping anchors to the lower
leg. These should start low and work upwards
but they must not wrap around the muscle
belly of the calf (See Diagram A).

SUPPORT TECHNIQUE- Using 1 1/2" white adhesive tape, apply one stirrup
starting on the inside upper anchor and finishing on
the outside upper anchor (See Diagram B).
- Apply one " U " strip starting on the inside mid-arch
anchor and finishing on the outside mid-arch anchor
(See Diagram B).

12

- Repeat the above steps two more times. Alternate the stirrups (moving forward) with the " U " strips (moving upward), in each case overlapping by half the width of the tape (See Diagram C).

" FIGURE 8 "
- Using 1 1/2" white adhesive tape, start the " figure 8 " support strip on the inside of the ankle, just above the malleolus (See Diagram D). Travel around the back, across the front, continuing down the inside of the ankle and under the foot (See Diagram E).
- Continue by pulling up on the outside, across the front and around the back to finish on the front of the ankle (See Diagram F). Make sure to tear the tape after completing the " figure 8 ."

HEEL LOCKS
- The first heel lock starts on the inside of the ankle just above the malleolus (See Diagram G).
- Continue behind the ankle, across the front, down the inside, under the foot and pull up on the outside of the heel (See Diagram H).
- The second heel lock continues from behind, travels across the front, down the outside, under the foot and pulls up on the inside of the heel (See Diagrams I & J).
- Finish the second heel lock on the front of the ankle (See Diagram K).

CLOSURES
- Begin closure of the lower leg starting just above the malleolus and working upwards. Overlap each strip by half the width of the tape and follow the leg contours (See Diagram L).
- Apply a finishing forefoot closure to seal the ends of all the " U " strips. Spread the toes apart before securing this piece (See Diagram L).

N.B. For an eversion sprain apply four to five stirrups, using a neutral force (ie., the pull is equal on each side of the ankle). Then apply double heel locks without the " figure 8 " strips. Once this is done, close the tape job.

13

ANKLE TAPE-CLOSED GIBNEY BASKETWEAVE

OUTSIDE VIEW

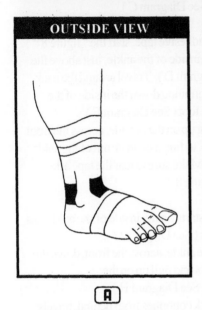

A

INSIDE & OUTSIDE VIEW

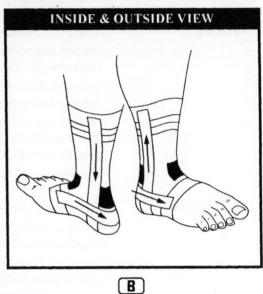

B

INSIDE & OUTSIDE VIEW

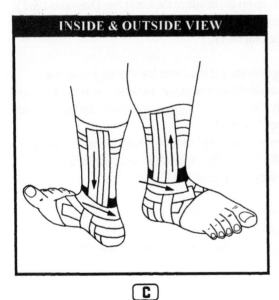

C

FRONT VIEW

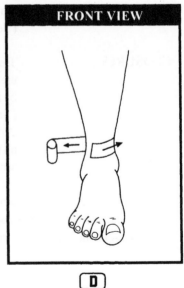

D

ANKLE TAPE-CLOSED GIBNEY BASKETWEAVE

FRONT VIEW
FIGURE 8

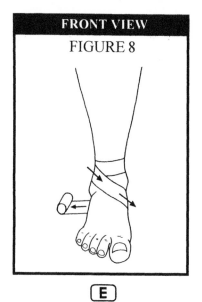

E

FRONT & OUTSIDE VIEW

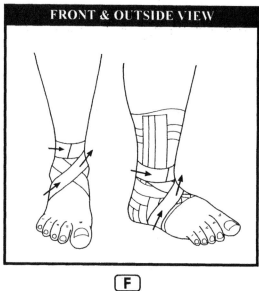

F

FRONT VIEW
HEEL LOCKS

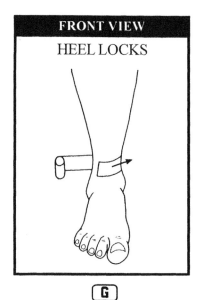

G

FRONT & OUTSIDE VIEW

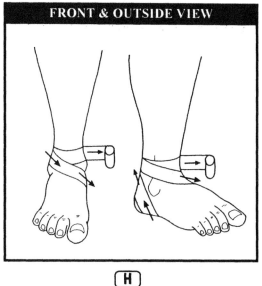

H

15

ANKLE TAPE-CLOSED GIBNEY BASKETWEAVE

FRONT & INSIDE VIEW

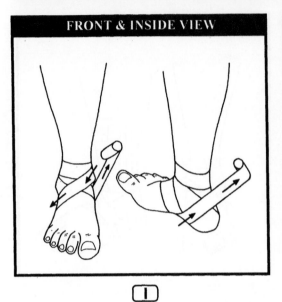

☐ I ☐

OUTSIDE VIEW

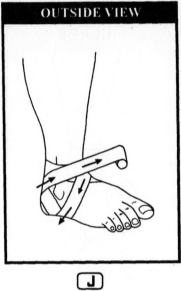

☐ J ☐

OUTSIDE VIEW

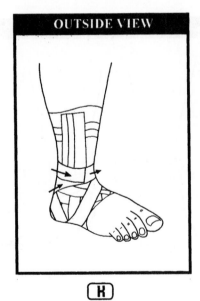

☐ H ☐

OUTSIDE VIEW

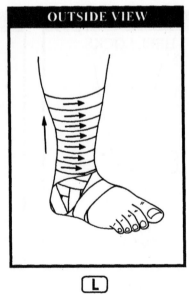

☐ L ☐

16

ANKLE TAPE-CLOSED GIBNEY (OPTION)

PURPOSE: - To substantially increase stability of the lateral ligaments by reducing the chance of an inversion sprain. This technique is useful with heavy individuals.

SUPPLIES: - tuf-skin spray
- 1 1/2" white adhesive tape
- skin lubricant
- 3" non tearing elastic tape
- heel & lace pads
- underwrap

IMPORTANT TEACHING POINTS:
SKIN PREPARATION
    AND
BODY POSITIONING - The foot is positioned so that the toes point upward (dorsiflexion).
- Spray the ankle with tuf-skin and place the lubricated heel & lace pads on the front and back of the ankle.
- Secure the heel & lace pads with underwrap.

ANCHORS - Using 3" non tearing elastic tape, apply one 3" anchor above the belly of the calf muscle (See Diagram A). Do not apply too much tension.
- Apply three 1 1/2" white adhesive tape anchors to the lower leg just below the belly of the calf muscle (See Diagram A). Overlap these three strips by half the width of the tape.
- Apply a 1 1/2" white adhesive tape anchor to the mid-arch area. Spread the toes apart before securing this arch anchor. Do not apply too much tension.

17

STIRRUPS

- Apply a 3" non tearing elastic tape strip starting on the inside of the ankle, level with the white adhesive tape anchors (See Diagram B).
- Continue downwards, under the foot and then pull up laterally to secure the stirrup on the upper 3" elastic tape anchor (See Diagrams B & C).
- Repeat two more stirrups using 1 1/2" white adhesive tape strips, each overlapping the other (See Diagram D).

CLOSURES

- Close the stirrups with two 1 1/2" white adhesive tape strips placed on top of the elastic anchor (See Diagram D).
- Complete this option technique with a " figure 8 " and heel locks, then close the lower leg (Refer to the closed gibney basketweave tape job).

18

ANKLE TÅPE-CLOSED GIBNEY (OPTION)

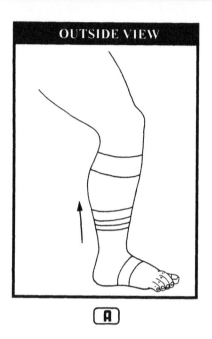

OUTSIDE VIEW

A

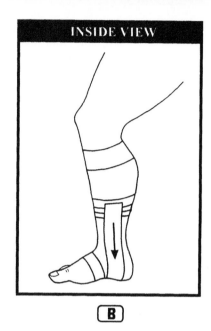

INSIDE VIEW

B

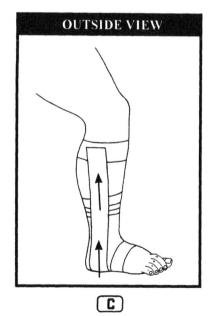

OUTSIDE VIEW

C

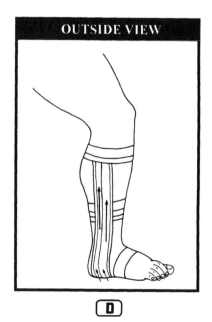

OUTSIDE VIEW

D

COTTON-ANKLE WRAP (LOUISIANA)

PURPOSE: - To prevent inversion sprains using an economical, washable and re-usable cloth ankle wrap.

SUPPLIES: - tuf-skin spray
- baby powder
- 2 " cloth wrap
- 1" or 1 1/2" white adhesive tape

IMPORTANT TEACHING POINTS:
SKIN PREPARATION
AND
BODY POSITIONING   - Position the ankle with the toes pointed upward (dorsiflexion).
- Apply tuf-skin to the front and back of the ankle.
- Cover the front and back of the ankle with baby powder to prevent friction.
- Place an athletic sock on the ankle.
- To establish the length of the ankle wrap, measure the distance from the floor to the palm above the athlete's head. Cut the wrap to this length. (approx. 8ft.)

SUPPORT TECHNIQUE
STARTING POSITION   - Make sure to use steady tension on the ankle wrap roll to avoid any wrinkles and open areas.
- Apply the cloth wrap on the inside of the ankle just above the malleolus. Go around once to secure the wrap into position (See Diagrams A & B).

"FIGURE 8"   - Coming from behind, start the " figure 8 " procedure by coming across the front, travelling on the inside of the ankle and under the foot (See Diagram C). Continue by pulling up on the outside, across the front, around the back and across the front again (See Diagrams D & E).

HEEL LOCKS

- The first of two heel locks follows next and continues from the inside of the ankle, under the foot and pulls up on the outside of the heel (See Diagram F).
- Continue with one complete revolution around the ankle, just above the malleolus (See Diagram G).
- Coming from behind once again, travel across the front, down the outside and under the foot (See Diagram H).
- For the second heel lock, travel on the inside of the heel and around the back continuing with one complete revolution (See Diagrams I & J) and finishing on the front of the ankle.
- Secure the ankle wrap with a small piece of 1 1/2" white adhesive tape to hold the tension (See Diagram K).

CLOSURES

- Repeat the entire procedure once with 1 1/2" white adhesive tape. Before securing the tape, fold the edge over to create a tab with which to remove the tape after the sport activity.

- To prevent the wrap ends from fraying, coat the two ends with nail polish or an oil base paint. Do not put the cloth into a clothes dryer after washing. Hang to dry.

COTTON-ANKLE WRAP (LOUISIANA)

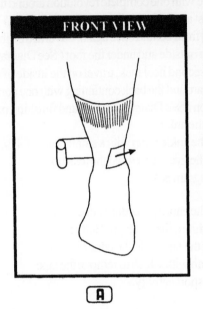

FRONT VIEW

A

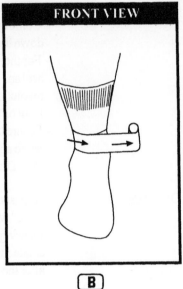

FRONT VIEW

B

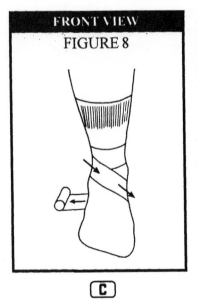

FRONT VIEW

FIGURE 8

C

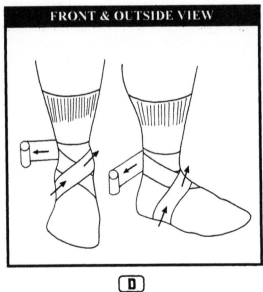

FRONT & OUTSIDE VIEW

D

COTTON-ANKLE WRAP (LOUISIANA)

HEEL LOCKS

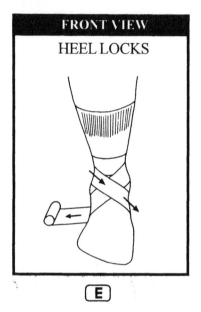

E

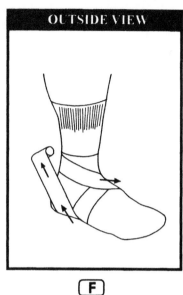

F

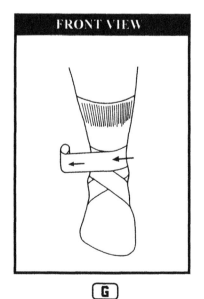

G

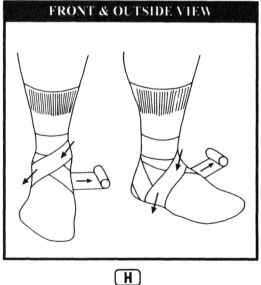

H

23

COTTON-ANKLE WRAP (LOUISIANA)

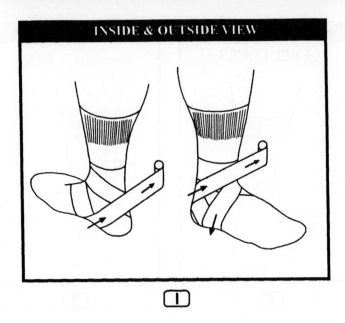
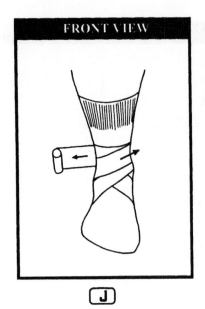
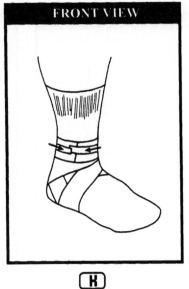
24

ANKLE TAPE-OPEN GIBNEY

PURPOSE: - To provide compression and stability to a sprained ankle
to assist with the healing process.

SUPPLIES: - tuf-skin spray
- horseshoe (felt or foam)
- 4" tensor bandage and clips
- 2" x 2" gauze pads
- underwrap
- 1 1/2" white adhesive tape
- skin lubricant
- heel & lace pads

IMPORTANT TEACHING POINTS:
SKIN PREPARATION
AND
BODY POSITIONING

- Position the ankle in a painfree position with the toes
pointing upward (dorsiflexion).
- Spray the ankle with tuf-skin.
- Apply a lubricated heel & lace pad to the front and
one to the back of the ankle (See Diagram A).
- Apply underwrap to the skin above the lateral and
medial malleolus, then apply underwrap to the
mid-forefoot using a " figure 8 ."
- Place a horseshoe pad on the injured side
of the ankle (See Diagram A).

ANCHORS

- Using 1 1/2" white adhesive tape, apply one
anchor to the mid-forefoot (do not close).
- Apply three anchors to the lower leg, overlapping by
half the width of the tape (See Diagram B).
Do not apply the anchors to the calf muscle.

25

SUPPORT TECHNIQUE- Using 1 1/2" white adhesive tape, apply one stirrup starting on the inside upper anchor and finishing on the outside upper anchor (See Diagram C). Apply one " U " strip starting on the inside mid-forefoot anchor and finishing on the outside mid-forefoot anchor (See Diagram C). Repeat the above steps two more times. Move the stirrups forward, overlapping by half the width of the tape and move the " U " strips upward, overlapping by half the width of the tape (See Diagram D).

- Apply two half heel locks to the inside of the ankle and two half heel locks to the outside of the ankle (See Diagram E).

CLOSURES

- Using 1 1/2" white adhesive tape, close the forefoot heel area and lower leg with overlapping " U " strips. Make sure to cover all stirrups (See Diagram F). By starting at the toes and working upward the swelling is forced out of the ankle.
- Seal both inside and outside edges, in each case using one continuous 1 1/2" white adhesive tape strip starting at the top and working down to the mid-forefoot (See Diagram G)
- Apply one closure strip to the mid-forefoot and one closure strip just below the calf (See Diagram H).
- Place a 2" x 2" gauze pad (folded in half) between each toe to prevent swelling to this area.
- Wrap a 4" tensor bandage around the ankle, starting at the toes, continuing upwards using a " figure 8 " spiral and finishing just below the calf (See Diagram I).
- Do not allow the athlete to wear the tensor while sleeping.
- Icing can be accomplished by placing the ankle (minus tensor) in a plastic bag then immersing the ankle in an ice bath. Protect the toes with a sock before the ice bath.
- Contact your doctor or therapist for appropriate icing instructions.

N.B. For an eversion sprain apply the same amount of stirrups, using a neutral force ie. the pull on the stirrups is equal on each side of the ankle.

ANKLE TAPE-OPEN GIBNEY

OUTSIDE VIEW

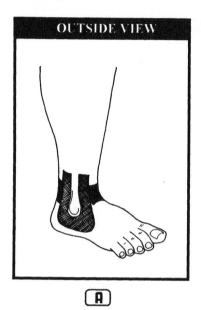

A

OUTSIDE VIEW

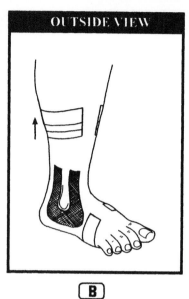

B

INSIDE & OUTSIDE VIEW

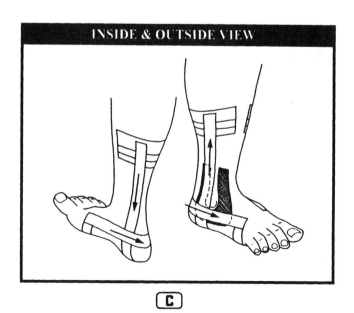

C

ANKLE TAPE-OPEN GIBNEY

INSIDE & OUTSIDE VIEW

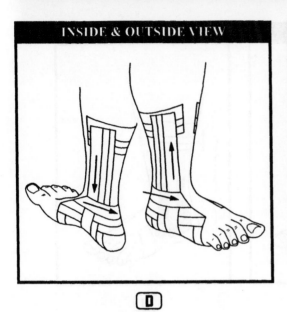

D

OUTSIDE VIEW

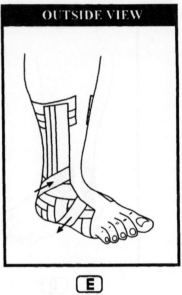

E

INSIDE & OUTSIDE VIEW

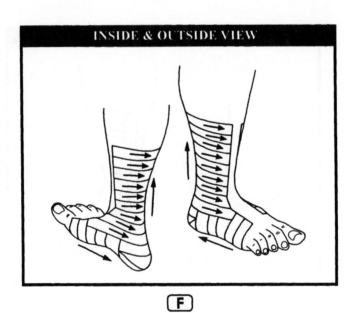

F

ANKLE TAPE-OPEN GIBNEY

INSIDE & OUTSIDE VIEW

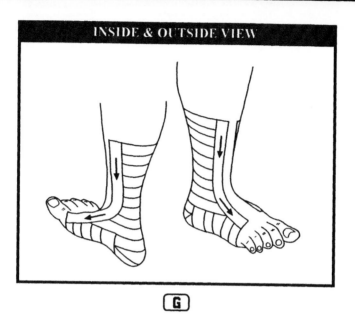

G

INSIDE & OUTSIDE VIEW

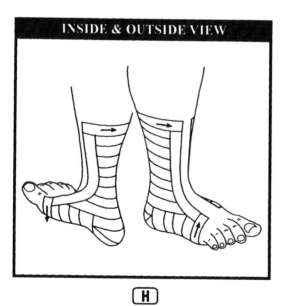

H

OUTSIDE VIEW

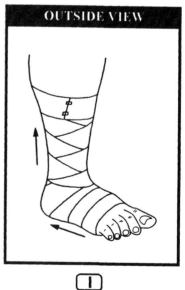

I

ACUTE ANKLE WRAP

PURPOSE: - To limit range of motion and provide compression for acute ankle sprains.

SUPPLIES: - underwrap (optional)
- 3" or 4" tensor bandage
- extended horseshoe made from 1/4" or 3/8" foam or felt
- 1 1/2" white adhesive tape

IMPORTANT TEACHING POINTS:
SKIN PREPARATION
AND
BODY POSITIONING - The foot is positioned so that the toes point upward. The ankle should be in as much dorsiflexion as tolerated.
- Place the extended horseshoe on the lateral aspect of the ankle (See Diagram A). For added compression, a second horseshoe may be placed on the medial aspect of the ankle. Hold the extended horseshoe(s) in place with underwrap (optional).

SUPPORT TECHNIQUE- The tensor bandage should start on the dorsum of the foot as close to the toes as possible. Spiral the bandage around the foot, two or three revolutions, overlapping each by half (See Diagrams B, C, D, E).
- Begin the first " figure 8 " by travelling around the back of the heel, keeping as low as possible (See Diagram F).
- Repeat this motion, overlapping the previous " figure 8 " by half. Continue this " herring bone " pattern up the leg. Finish approximately 6" above the maleoli (See Diagrams G, H, I, J). Secure the bandage with clips.

30

- Additional " figure 8 " strips can be added with 1 1/2" white adhesive tape to help keep the foot in dorsiflexion. This position allows for the least amount of swelling in the joint space.
- The tensor bandage and horseshoe(s) should be removed prior to applying ice.
- The bandage should not be worn while sleeping.

NOTE

- The athlete may need to stay off the ankle until seen by a physician, crutches are suggested.

ACUTE ANKLE WRAP

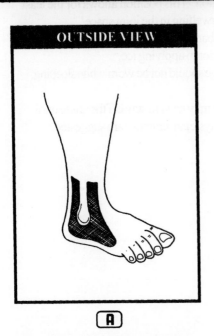

OUTSIDE VIEW

A

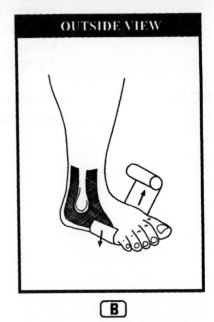

OUTSIDE VIEW

B

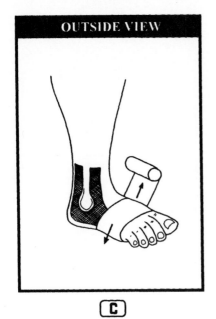

OUTSIDE VIEW

C

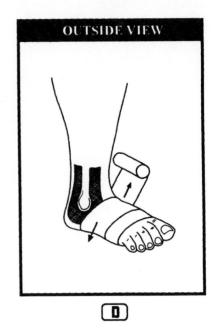

OUTSIDE VIEW

D

ACUTE ANKLE WRAP

OUTSIDE VIEW

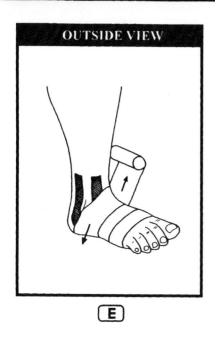

E

OUTSIDE VIEW

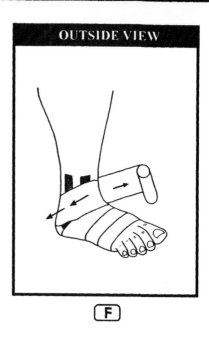

F

OUTSIDE VIEW

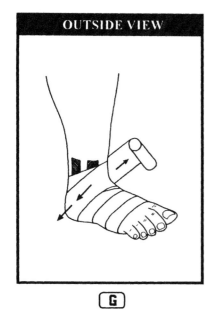

G

OUTSIDE VIEW

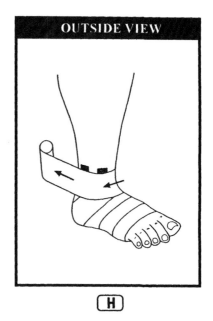

H

ACUTE ANKLE WRAP

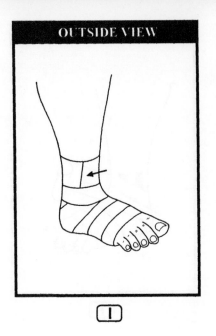

I

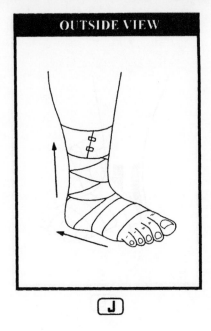

J

34

CHAPTER TWO

BUNION (HALLUX VALGUS)

TURF TOE

ARCH TAPING-PLANTAR FASCITIS

MOLESKIN ARCH TAPING

ACHILLES TENDON TAPING

"SHIN SPLINTS" LATERAL COMPARTMENT

"SHIN SPLINTS" MEDIAL COMPARTMENT

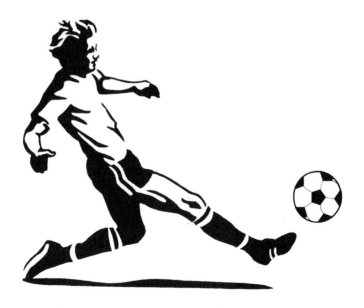

BUNION (HALLUX VALGUS)

PURPOSE: - To reduce valgus stress on the big toe (MTP- metatarsal phalangeal joint). (See Diagram A).

SUPPLIES: - 1" and 1 1/2" white adhesive tape
- one small band-aid
- tuf-skin spray

IMPORTANT TEACHING POINTS:

SKIN PREPARATION
- Shave the big toe and forefoot if necessary.
- Spray the big toe and forefoot with tuf-skin.
- Cover the big toe nail with a band-aid to prevent trauma.

ANCHORS
- Using 1 1/2" white adhesive tape, apply two forefoot anchors to the middle of the arch (See Diagram B) and be sure to spread apart the toes before securing this piece.
- Using 1" white adhesive tape, apply two anchors to the big toe and overlap each by half the width of the tape (See Diagram B). Do not apply too much tension.

SUPPORT TECHNIQUE
- Pull the big toe in the opposite direction from the bunion position (See Diagram C).
- Apply three 1" white adhesive tape strips starting on the inside (medial side) of the big toe while pulling down towards the arch anchor. These strips should overlap each other by half the width of the tape (See Diagram C).

CLOSURES

- Using 1" white adhesive tape, apply two closing strips around the big toe and overlap these strips by half the width of the tape (See Diagram D).
- If the desired tension on the support strips is inadequate at this time, detach the strips at the forefoot anchor and re-apply the tension. Secure the strips in place again.
- Apply two final 1 1/2" closures over the mid-arch area and spread the toes before securing the strip (See Diagram D).
- Be sure the support strips do not extend past the anchors as it will make closures difficult.
- Placing a foam pad between the big toe and the second toe may add to comfort.

BUNION (HALLUX VALGUS)

BOTTOM VIEW

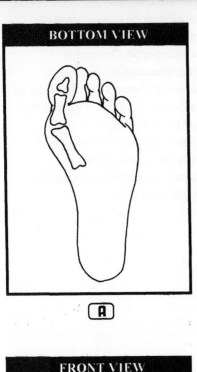

A

FRONT VIEW

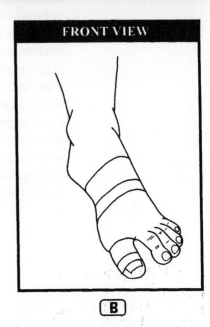

B

FRONT VIEW

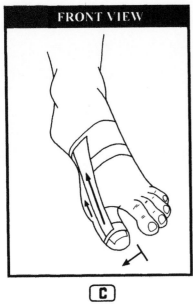

C

FRONT VIEW

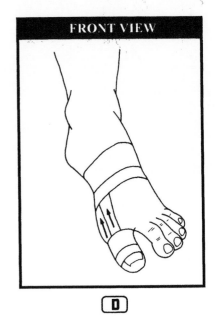

D

TURF TOE

PURPOSE: - To prevent excessive hyperextension of the MTP joint.

SUPPLIES: - tuf-skin spray
- 1" white adhesive tape
- 1 1/2" white adhesive tape

IMPORTANT TEACHING POINTS:
SKIN PREPARATION
   AND
BODY POSITIONING - The big toe should be in a neutral position.
- Shave excess hair off of the top of the forefoot and big toe.
- Spray the forefoot and the big toe with tuf-skin.

ANCHORS - Apply one 1" white adhesive tape anchor around the big toe (See Diagram A). If the big toe is long, use two anchor strips. Not too tight!
- Using 1 1/2" white adhesive tape, apply two arch anchors to the mid-arch area (See Diagrams A & B). Spread the toes apart by pushing upwards with your fingers before securing these anchor strips. This will assimilate weight bearing on the foot.

CHECK REIN - Measure the distance from the arch anchors to the toe anchor. On the middle of the big toe, attach one 1" strip of white adhesive tape with three 1" " X " strips on top of it to create a checkrein. The ends of the checkrein must be narrow enough to fit on the big toe (See Diagram C). The " X " must cross over the MP Joint line. Wiggle the toes to be sure.

CLOSURES

- Close the big toe with one 1" white adhesive tape strip (See Diagram D).
- Close the mid arch of the forefoot with two 1 1/2" white adhesive strips. Spread the toes apart prior to securing the closures (See Diagram D). If the big toe is very long, two or three closure strips may be necessary.

NOTE

- This support technique can be done on the dorsum of the foot to prevent hyper-flexion.

40

TURF TOE

BOTTOM VIEW

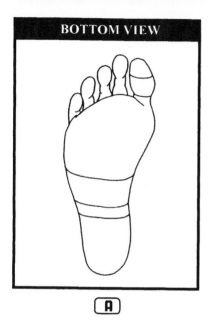

A

SIDE VIEW

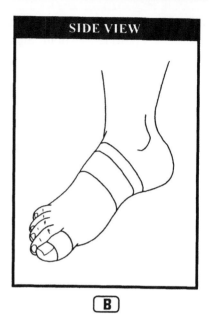

B

BOTTOM VIEW

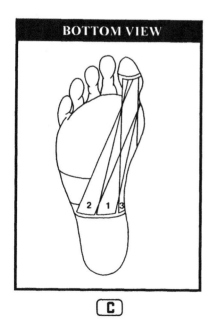

C

BOTTOM VIEW

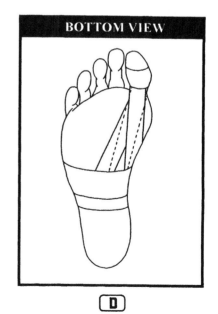

D

41

ARCH TAPING-PLANTAR FASCITIS

PURPOSE: - Used to support the plantar fascia (arch) and can also
provide relief from " Shin Splints " by increasing
shock absortion in the foot.

SUPPLIES: - tuf-skin spray
- heel & lace pads
- skin lubricant
- 1 " white adhesive tape
- 1 1/2" white adhesive tape
- 2" white adhesive tape

IMPORTANT TEACHING POINTS:

SKIN PREPARATION - Spray the top and bottom of the foot with
tuf-skin.
- Place half of a lubricated heel & lace pad at the
back of the heel and secure it in place
with one 2" white adhesive tape strip
(See Diagram A).

ANCHORS - Position the foot in dorsiflexion with the
toes curled. This accentuates the arch
(not shown in Diagram).
- Apply one forefoot anchor at the base
of the toes using 1 1/2" white adhesive
tape (See Diagram A). Before securing
this strip spread the athlete's toes apart
with your fist.
- Apply one 1 1/2" peripheral anchor strip by
starting on the outside forefoot anchor,
continuing around the heel and finishing on the
inside of the forefoot anchor (See Diagram B).

42

SUPPORT TECHNIQUE - These support strips require 1" white adhesive tape.
- Start the first arch strip on the forefoot anchor beneath the fourth toe. Carry this strip down and over the heel pad to finish at the base of the big toe (See Diagram C).
- Repeat the arch strip twice more by having the strip start on the forefoot anchor beneath the 3rd and 2nd toes respectively. These strips should finish near the base of the big toe (See Diagrams D & E).

CLOSURES
- Begin closure of the arch support strips by using 1 1/2" white adhesive tape.
- Begin the first closure strip just in front of the heel by starting and finishing the strip on the top of the foot (See Diagram F).
- Continue to apply these closure strips, working down towards the toes. In each case, the strips must start on the outside of the top of the foot and then pull up on the inside arch to finish on top of the foot.
- Be sure to spread apart the toes before securing the tape strips.
- All the toes should be free to move so do not cover them up.

ARCH TAPING-PLANTAR FASCITIS

SIDE VIEW

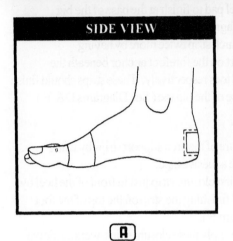

A

SIDE VIEW

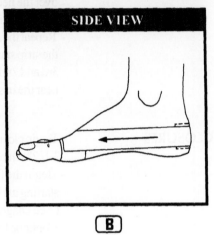

B

BOTTOM VIEW

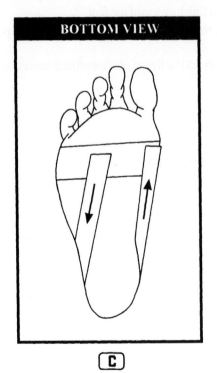

C

BOTTOM VIEW

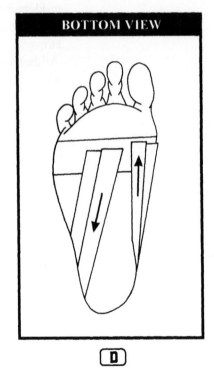

D

44

ARCH TAPING-PLANTAR FASCITIS

BOTTOM VIEW

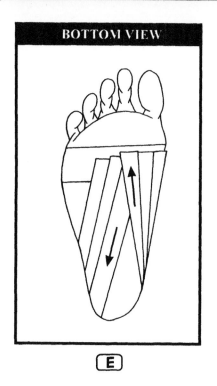

E

BOTTOM VIEW

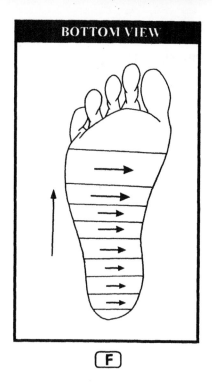

F

45

PURPOSE: - To provide support to the arch and to the foot.

SUPPLIES: - 3" moleskin
- tuf-skin spray
- 1 1/2" white adhesive tape

IMPORTANT TEACHING POINTS:
SKIN PREPARATION
    AND
BODY POSITIONING - Spray the bottom of the foot with tuf-skin.
- Have the athlete sit on a taping table
with his/her arch facing the person applying the tape.
- The arch should be relaxed.

ANCHORS - Using 1 1/2" white adhesive tape, secure an anchor
around the forefoot near the base of the toes. Be sure
to spread apart the toes by pushing on the bottom of the
foot. This will ensure that the anchor does not
interfere with the normal movements while
the athlete is weight bearing (See Diagram A).

SUPPORT TECHNIQUE- Once the moleskin has been measured and
cut (See Diagram B) secure it at the back of
the heel then along the length of the forefoot
anchor (See Diagrams A & C).

CLOSURES - Begin closure of the arch by using 1 1/2" strips
of white adhesive tape. These should start
on the outside of the foot and then pull
up on the inside of the arch. The first
closure starts just beyond the mid-arch area.
Continue to overlap the closure strips
by half the width of the tape until the forefoot
anchor is reached (See Diagram D).

MOLESKIN ARCH TAPING

BACK VIEW

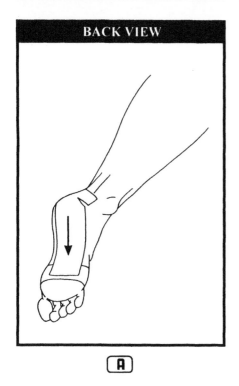

A

MOLESKIN

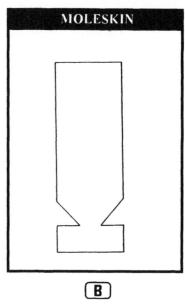

B

SIDE VIEW

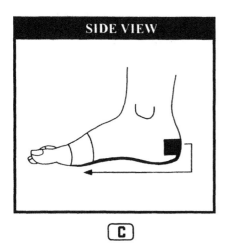

C

SIDE VIEW

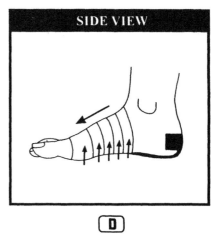

D

47

ACHILLES TENDON TAPING

PURPOSE: - To provide support for the achilles tendon by limiting extreme dorsiflexion of the ankle.

SUPPLIES:
- tuf-skin spray
- 3" non tearing elastic tape
- skin lubricant
- 1 1/2" white adhesive tape
- medium density foam
- 3" elastic tape (very thin)

IMPORTANT TEACHING POINTS:
SKIN PREPARATION
AND
BODY POSITIONING
- Shave the lower leg.
- Apply tuf-skin spray to the lower leg.
- Position the athlete lying on his/her stomach on a table or kneeling on a chair with toes slightly pointed (plantar flexion). Too much plantar flexion predisposes the athlete to inversion ankle sprains.

ANCHORS
- Apply two 1 1/2" white adhesive tape forefoot anchors to the mid-arch and overlap them by half the width of the tape. Spread apart the toes before securing each strip (See Diagram A).
- Apply three or four 1 1/2" white adhesive tape strips to the lower leg just below the belly of the calf. Overlap these strips by half the width of the tape. For athletes with long lower legs and high calf muscles, do not position these anchors more than twelve inches above the heel (See Diagram A).

SUPPORT TECHNIQUE - Lay a 3" non tearing elastic tape strip on the bottom of the forefoot anchor. Secure this with a 1 1/2" white adhesive tape strip (See Diagram B). Pull up the non tearing elastic tape strip while applying tension and secure it to the calf anchors with a 1 1/2" white adhesive tape strip (See Diagram B).

48

- Lay a second strip of 3" non tearing elastic tape on the plantar aspect of the forefoot. Secure this with a 1 1/2" white adhesive tape strip.
- Measure this piece so that it is long enough to be split and secured to the calf anchor (See Diagram B).

CLOSURES
- Close the forefoot with two 1 1/2" white adhesive tape strips. Overlap these by half the width of the tape (See Diagram C).
- Close the lower leg with five or six 1 1/2" white adhesive tape strips. Do not apply the closures to the calf muscle belly as it could cramp or fatigue. Overlap the closures by half the width of the tape (See Diagram C). Have the athlete contract the calf by pointing the toes into your thigh.

N.B. Fold the elastic tape over on each side of the base of the achilles tendon and then apply skin lubricant to the achilles tendon to stop any friction.

A heel lift may be used (medium density foam) to give support to the achilles. It is a good idea for the athlete to wear one heel lift in each shoe to prevent any biomechanical imbalances.

OPTIONAL CLOSURE
- Spiral a very thin piece of 3" elastic tape around the entire procedure from the forefoot upwards to secure the finished technique (See Diagram D for closure).

OPTION
- Additional heel locks and stirrups followed by closures will decrease the risk of ankle sprains.

ACHILLES TENDON TAPING

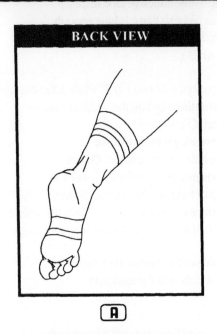

A

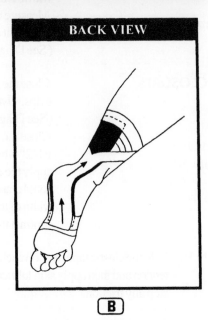

B

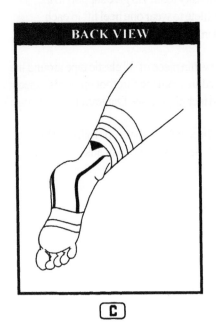

C

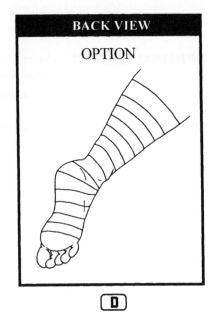

OPTION

D

50

"SHIN SPLINTS" LATERAL COMPARTMENT

PURPOSE: - To provide support to the outside (lateral) muscles of the lower leg due to pain from overuse of the limb.

SUPPLIES: - tuf-skin spray
  - 1 1/2" white adhesive tape
  - 3/ 8 " or 1/4" thick foam pad

IMPORTANT TEACHING POINTS:
SKIN PREPARATION
  AND
BODY POSITIONING - Shave the lower leg.
  - Spray the lower leg with tuf-skin.
  - Have the athlete stand on a table.
  - Place a small pad 1" wide and 6" long over the area of tenderness. The use of 3/ 8" or 1/ 4" thick foam is ideal (See Diagram A).

ANCHORS - Place one 1 1/ 2" white adhesive tape anchor on the outside of the lower leg. This piece starts at the tip of the lateral malleolus and rises up the lower leg to just below the muscle belly of the calf (See Diagram A).
  - Place another 1 1/ 2" white adhesive tape anchor on the inside of the lower leg. The boundaries for this strip lie between the tip of the medial malleolus and just below the calf muscle belly (See Diagram A).

SUPPORT TECHNIQUE- Begin the spiral support strips on the inside of the lower leg, just above the medial malleolus (See Diagram B). These strips start on the inside anchor, travel behind the achilles tendon, spiral up and over the area of tenderness and finish on the inside anchor (See Diagram B).

51

- Overlap the spiral support strips by half the width of the tape.
- Repeat the spiral technique about three to four times. The number of strips will depend on the length of the lower leg.

CLOSURES
- Start the 1 1/2" white adhesive tape closure strips just above the lateral and medial malleolus. All closure strips start on the inside, travel down on an angle to pass around the achilles and then rise back up on an angle. Tear off the strips of tape at this point. Repeat this "angle down" and "angle up" procedure until the support technique is closed in. This will create a "herring bone" pattern (See Diagram C).
- Do not tape over the muscle belly of the calf as the muscle could cramp or fatigue.

OPTION
- For extra support and shock absorption, use the arch taping procedure in combination with the shin splint tape job.

"SHIN SPLINTS" LATERAL COMPARTMENT

FRONT VIEW

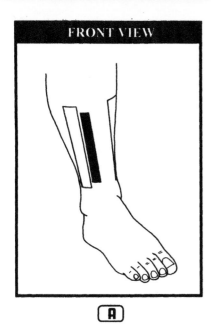

A

FRONT VIEW

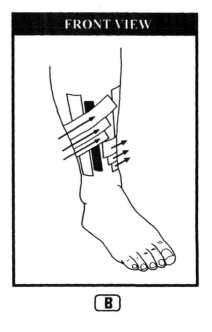

B

FRONT VIEW

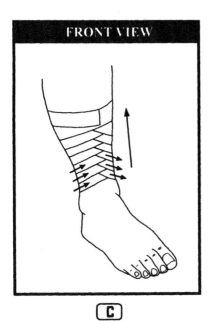

C

"SHIN SPLINTS" MEDIAL COMPARTMENT

SPECIAL INSTRUCTIONS

PURPOSE

- To provide support to the inside muscles
of the lower leg due to pain from overuse
of the limb.

SKIN PREPARATION

- Same taping materials as lateral compartment.
- Move the compression pad to the inside of
the lower leg.

SUPPORT TECHNIQUE

- These strips start on the outside of the lower leg
then spiral upwards moving medially.

CLOSURES

- These begin on the outside of the lower leg.
They traverse downward on the outside of the
lower leg and finish by pulling up and
over the inside of the lower leg.

CHAPTER THREE

KNEE-MEDIAL COLLATERAL LIGAMENT

KNEE (HYPEREXTENSION)

PATELLA TENDON TAPING

PATELLA STABILIZING SUPPORT

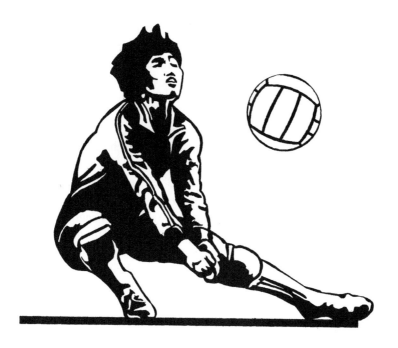

KNEE-MEDIAL COLLATERAL LIGAMENT

PURPOSE: - To provide support for a medial collateral ligament.

SUPPLIES: - 2" & 3" elastic tape   - heel & lace pad
            - underwrap   - skin lubricant
            - 1 1/2" white adhesive tape   - tuf-skin spray

IMPORTANT TEACHING POINTS:
SKIN PREPARATION
    AND
BODY POSITIONING - Shave the thigh and lower leg.
- Spray the entire thigh, knee and calf with tuf-skin.
- Apply a lubricated heel & lace pad to the back of the knee to prevent irritation.
- Secure the heel & lace pad with underwrap starting just above the calf and finishing mid-thigh. The underwrap will be secured by the elastic anchors.
- Position the athlete by placing a 1 1/2" roll of white adhesive tape under the heel (See Diagram A).
- Once the leg is bent (15 degrees), internally rotate the lower leg so that the toes face inward.

ANCHORS
- Have the athlete contract both the calf and thigh when applying these anchors.
- Apply the upper anchors mid to upper thigh using two or three 3" elastic tape strips. These should be overlapped by half the width and must be applied directly to the skin (See Diagram B). The first strip should be above the belly of the hamstrings.
- Apply two 3" elastic tape anchors just below the mid-calf and overlap each strip by half the width of the tape. These strips must be applied to the skin (See Diagram B).

56

SUPPORT TECHNIQUE - Use 2" elastic tape to apply the following support strips.

- Start the first support strip on the outside of the lower anchor (See Diagram C).
- This strip should traverse upwards crossing the joint line but remaining below the knee cap. The tape must be stretched to the maximum and then secured to the upper anchors.
- The second support strip starts on the inner part of the calf anchors. It crosses the joint line, but rises above the knee cap. The tape must be stretched to the maximum and then secured to the upper anchors (See Diagram D).
- The third strip travels on the inside of the knee travelling from the calf anchor to the upper thigh anchors. Slightly stretch this tape strip (See Diagram E).
- Repeat the above support techniques with 1 1/2" white adhesive tape. Fold the white tape at the joint line to reinforce.

DE-ROTATION STRIPS

- Always verify placement of strips as they cross over the joint line.
- Using 2" elastic tape, start the de-rotation strip at the calf anchor on the front of the lower leg. Pull the strip inwards and spiral upwards behind the knee, then upwards around the outside of the thigh to finish on the upper inner thigh anchor (See Diagram F).

CLOSURES

- Close the lower leg using 3" elastic tape strips. Start at the calf anchor and then work upwards to below the knee cap. Do not spiral continuously. Cut the tape after each turn around the leg and overlap the pieces by half the width. Continue the closure above the knee and then finish on the upper thigh (See Diagram G).

- Be sure never to end your tape on the inside of the thigh, this will result in the tape rolling off due to friction of the other thigh.
- Use one 6" tensor bandage or one double length 6" tensor bandage to secure the 3" elastic tape closures. Make sure the tensor bandage starts at the calf and works up to the top of the thigh. The tensor bandage should cover the entire leg. Secure the tensor bandage at the upper thigh with one or two 3" elastic tape strips.

KNEE-MEDIAL COLLATERAL LIGAMENT

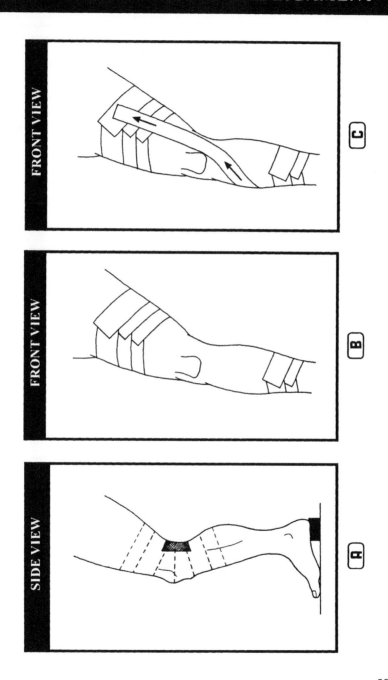

FRONT VIEW **C**

FRONT VIEW **B**

SIDE VIEW **A**

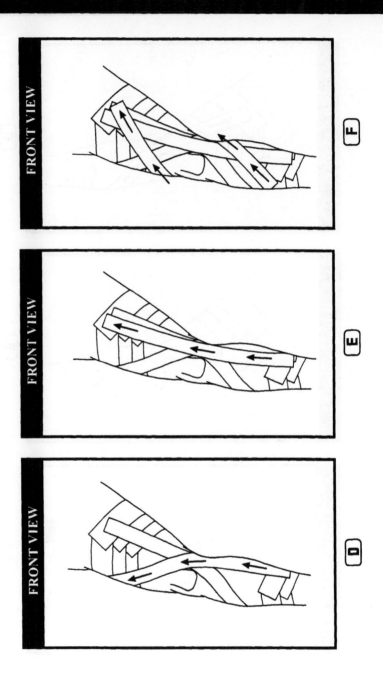

KNEE-MEDIAL COLLATERAL LIGAMENT

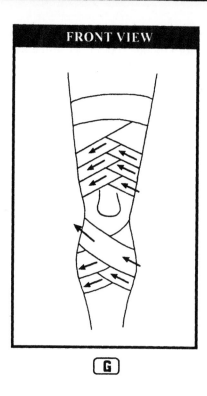

FRONT VIEW

G

KNEE (HYPEREXTENSION)

PURPOSE: - To prevent hyperextension of the knee in order to provide support for a sprained posterior capsule, a lax anterior cruciate ligament or strained lower hamstring tendons.

SUPPLIES:
- 3" elastic tape
- skin lubricant
- tuf-skin spray
- 1 1/2" white adhesive tape
- underwrap
- heel & lace pad
- 6" tensor bandages (2), or one double length

IMPORTANT TEACHING POINTS:
SKIN PREPARATION
AND
BODY POSITIONING
- Shave the thigh and lower leg.
- Spray the entire calf & thigh with tuf-skin.
- Apply a lubricated heel & lace pad to the back of the knee to prevent irritation (See Diagram B).
- Secure the heel & lace pad with underwrap starting just above the calf and finishing mid-thigh.
- Position the limb by placing a roll of 1 1/2" white adhesive tape under the athlete's heel (See Diagram A).
- Have the athlete internally rotate his or her lower leg so that the toes face inward.

ANCHORS
- Apply two or three 3" elastic tape anchors to the upper thigh and overlap each one by half the width of the tape. Be sure to have the athlete contract the thigh muscles (See Diagram B).
- Apply two or three 3 " elastic tape anchors around the lower leg (See Diagram B).
- Position the first strip below the belly of the calf and the second one mid-belly.
- These strips should overlap each other by half the width of the tape. Have the athlete contract the calf muscles before securing these strips.

62

CHECKREIN
FORMATION

- Measure the distance from one anchor to another by using the white adhesive tape (See Diagram C). Lay this strip on a table and add four more to it to create a fan shaped checkrein. Secure a 1 1/2" white adhesive tape piece around the centre of the checkrein (See Diagram D).

CLOSURES

- Position the pre-formed checkrein on the back of the leg (See Diagram D). Secure the lower leg first with three 3" elastic tape strips (See Diagram E). Be sure to maintain at least 15 degrees of flexion.
- Now secure the checkrein on the thigh by using four 3" elastic tape closures. Overlap these strips by half the width of the tape (See Diagram E).
- Check the function of the tape job. If the checkrein is too loose, fold the center of the fan onto itself and then re-secure it with two strips of 3" elastic tape. Do not end these on the inside of the thigh.
- Use two 6" tensor bandages or one double length 6" tensor bandage to secure the 3" elastic tape closures. Make sure the tensor bandage(s) start at the calf and work up to the top of the thigh. The tensor bandage(s) should cover the entire leg. Secure the tensor bandage at the upper thigh with one or two 3" elastic tape strips.

OPTION CLOSURE

- To add more support to the knee-hyperextension technique, add the de-rotation strip as found in the knee-medial collateral ligament taping procedure (See de-rotation strips section). This de-rotation strip is applied immediately after the anchors. Then complete the knee-hyperextension technique as shown.

KNEE (HYPEREXTENSION)

SIDE VIEW

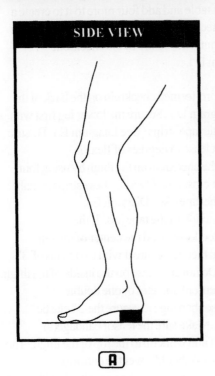

A

BACK VIEW

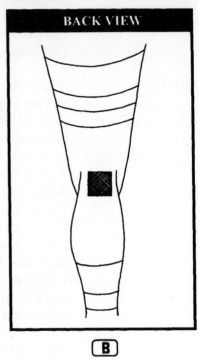

B

KNEE (HYPEREXTENSION)

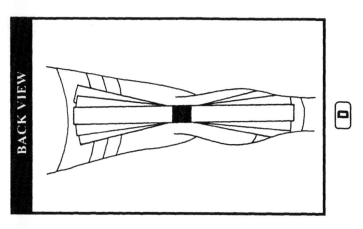

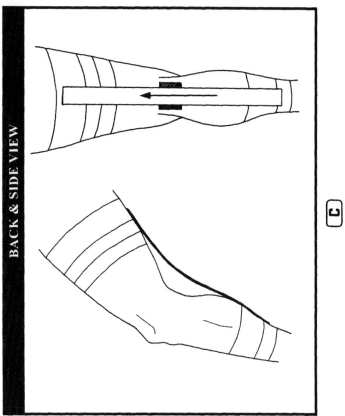

KNEE (HYPEREXTENSION)

BACK & SIDE VIEW

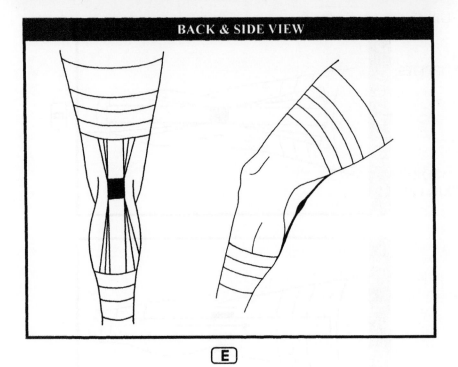

E

PATELLA TENDON TAPING

PURPOSE: - To provide support to the patella tendon and to take stress off the patella tendon insertion.

SUPPLIES: - 1 1/2" white adhesive tape or 2" elastic tape
- tuf-skin spray
- one heel & lace pad
- foam (3/8" thick x 1/2" wide x 2" long)
- skin lubricant

IMPORTANT TEACHING POINTS:

SKIN PREPARATION - Shave a small strip on the front and back of the knee on a horizontal line around the area of discomfort.
- Spray the front and back of the knee with tuf-skin.
- Cut the lubricated heel & lace pad in half and place the two sections behind the knee.

BODY POSITIONING - Position the athlete with the leg slightly bent, supporting the heel with a 1 1/2" roll of white adhesive tape (See Diagram A). For added pressure, passively place the knee in hyperextension, with quadriceps relaxed.

SUPPORT TECHNIQUE
&
CLOSURES
- Place the foam over the area of the tendon that requires support, just above the tibial tubercule (See Diagram B).
- Secure a 1 1/2" white adhesive tape strip around the patella tendon and the back of the knee. Place pressure on the anterior aspect of the knee but not on the posterior aspect of the knee (See Diagrams B & C).
- Repeat the horizontal closure piece again, then secure the strip on the front of the knee.
- Be sure the athlete can do a full squat and that the tape is not too tight.

67

PATELLA TENDON TAPING

SIDE VIEW

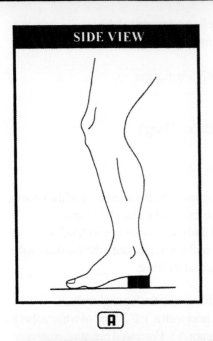

A

FRONT VIEW

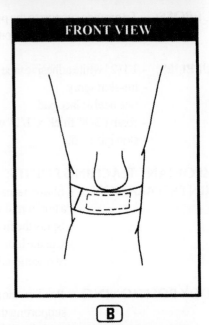

B

SIDE VIEW

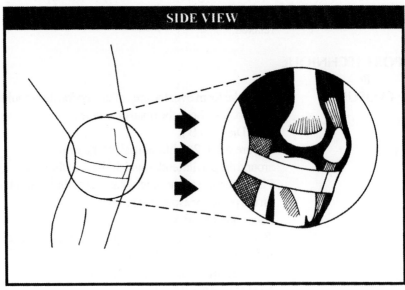

C

PATELLA STABILIZING SUPPORT

PURPOSE: - To prevent the patella from tracking laterally, subluxing or dislocating.

SUPPLIES: - 3" non tearing elastic tape
- tuf-skin spray, skin lubricant
- heel & lace pads
- 1 1/2" or 2" elastic tape
- 1 1/2" white adhesive tape
- 3/8" or 1/4" thick orthopedic felt or medium density foam (Horse Shoe Shape)

IMPORTANT TEACHING POINTS:
SKIN PREPARATION
AND
BODY POSITIONING - Shave the hair from just above and below the knee cap.
- Spray the front and back of the knee with tuf-skin.
- Position the athlete in a supported sitting position so that the quadriceps muscles are relaxed. Now place a small roll beneath the middle of the thigh (See Diagram A). This will allow you to access the back of the knee to complete the taping procedure.
- Place two lubricated heel and lace pads on the back of the knee for protection (See Diagram A).
- Place the horse shoe on the outside of the patella (See Diagram B).

SUPPORT TECHNIQUE- Create a patella stabilizing strip from 3" non tearing elastic tape by cutting one end of the tape into two equal sections. The cut should be about 6 " deep (See Diagram A). Place the 6 " split ends on the inside of the knee so that they surround the inside of the knee cap (See Diagram B).

69

- Roll the tape around the back of the knee, over the heel & lace pads and up to the lateral side of the knee cap (See Diagram B).
- Advance the elastic tape 6" beyond the outside edge of the knee cap and horse shoe then cut the tape (See Diagram B).
- Divide the end into two equal sections then cut them back to one inch beyond the outside edge of the horse shoe (See Diagram B).
- Move the lower strip upwards to be applied to the top of the knee cap. Move the upper strip downwards and secure below the knee cap (See Diagram C).
- This final step prevents the possibility of rips occuring along the seams.

CLOSURES

- Apply a continuous strip of 1 1/2" elastic tape that will cover the skin above the knee cap. This same strip must continue from the inside and outside of the thigh to cross down behind the knee (See Diagram D). This strip will eventually overlap on the patella tendon (See Diagram E).
- Add a 1 1/2" white adhesive tape strip horizontally below the knee cap to secure the continuous elastic " X " strip (See Diagram E).

PATELLA STABILIZING SUPPORT

SIDE LEG VIEW - HORSESHOE & TAPE STRIP

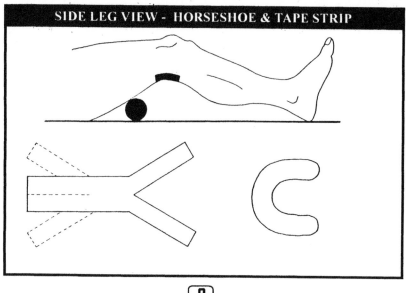

A

FRONT & SIDE VIEW

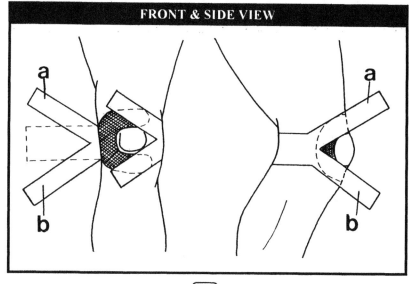

B

71

PATELLA STABILIZING SUPPORT

FRONT & SIDE VIEW

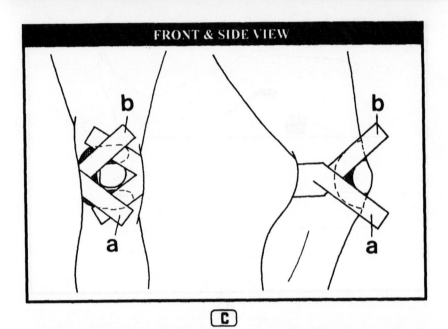

C

BACK VIEW

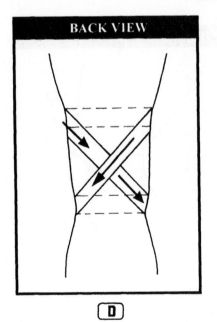

D

FRONT VIEW

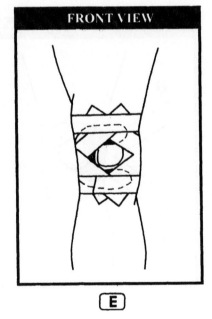

E

CHAPTER FOUR

QUADRICEPS SUPPORT

QUADRICEPS SUPPORT (OPTION)

HAMSTRING SUPPORT

HIP FLEXOR-GROIN WRAP

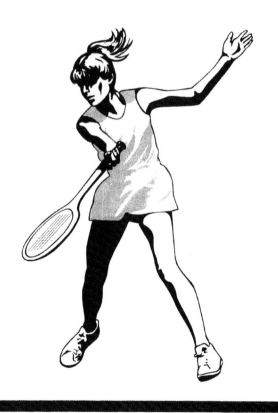

QUADRICEPS SUPPORT

PURPOSE: - To provide compression to a strain or a contusion to the quadriceps muscles in the acute stage.

SUPPLIES: - underwrap
- tuf-skin spray
- 6" tensor bandage
- 2" elastic tape
- pressure pad
- 1 1/2" white adhesive tape
- 2" white adhesive tape

IMPORTANT TEACHING POINTS:
SKIN PREPARATION
    AND
BODY POSITIONING - Position the athlete by placing a 1 1/2" roll of white adhesive tape under the heel (See Diagram A).
- Shave the hair from the front of the thigh.
- Spray the thigh with tuf-skin.
- Apply a pressure pad over the area of injury.

ANCHORS - Secure one 2" white adhesive tape strip on the outside of the thigh and one on the inside of the thigh (See Diagram B).

SUPPORT TECHNIQUE- Using 1 1/2" white adhesive tape, start the first support strip just below the area of injury on the inner thigh, moving upwards on a 45 degree angle (See Diagram C).
- The next support strip starts on the outside anchor on the front of the thigh. From here the strip travels upwards on a 45 degree angle.
- Repeat the strips while overlapping by half the width of the tape until the area is fully covered (See Diagram D).
- These support strips do not go entirely around the thigh (See Diagram E).
- Cover the support with underwrap. This decreases the possibility of the wrap moving or sliding during activity.

74

CLOSURES

- Close the entire tape job with a 6" tensor bandage or one 6" double length tensor bandage for large quadriceps.
- The athlete should contract the quadriceps during application.
- Start applying the tensor below the injury and then work upwards with a " TUG " on a 45 degree angle. Now spiral around the thigh and work the tensor downwards with a " TUG " on a 45 degree angle.
- Repeat the above procedure to create a herring bone pattern (See Diagram F).
- Secure the wrap with three clips. Do not finish the clips on the inside of the leg as they could rub and cut the opposite leg or just pop off. Secure the wrap with two or three 2" elastic tape strips, overlapping by half the tape width (See Diagram F).

QUADRICEPS SUPPORT

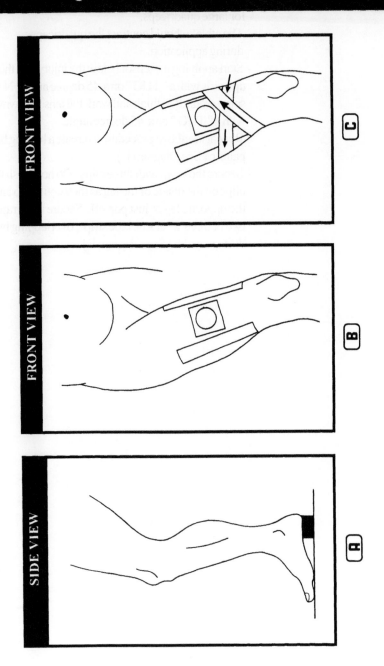

76

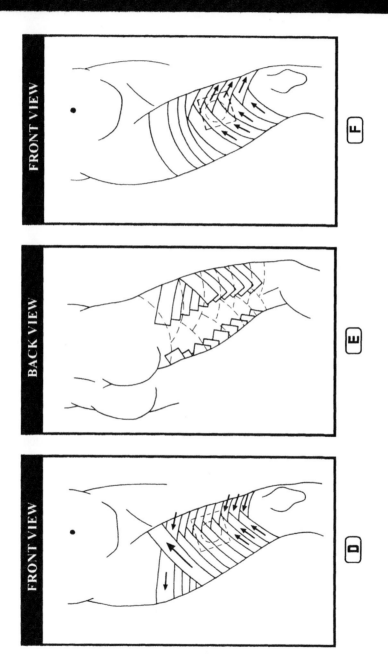

QUADRICEPS SUPPORT (OPTION)

PURPOSE: - To provide support to the quadriceps muscles.
This technique may be used as an option.

SUPPLIES: - tuf-skin spray
- underwrap
- 1 1/2" white adhesive tape
- 3" elastic tape
- 6" tensor bandage
- protective foam pad (medium density)

IMPORTANT TEACHING POINTS:
SKIN PREPARATION
    AND
BODY POSITIONING - Shave the front of the thigh.
- Apply the tuf-skin to the front and back of the thigh.
- The athlete should be positioned so that the knee is bent at approximately a 30 degree angle. Position the athlete by placing a 1 1/2" roll of white adhesive tape under the heel (See Diagram A).

SUPPORT TECHNIQUE- Apply four 1 1/2" white adhesive tape strips (rolled sticky side out) over the area to be protected (See Diagram B). These strips will help to prevent the foam pad and tensor bandage from sliding down the leg during activity.
- Apply a pad over the area to be protected (3/8" thick, medium density foam as a minimum requirement- See Diagram C).

78

CLOSURES

- Close the entire tape job with a 6" tensor bandage.
- Start applying the tensor below the area to be supported, then work upwards with a " TUG " on a 45 degree angle. Now spiral around the thigh and work the tensor downwards with a " TUG " on a 45 degree angle. Repeat this up and down configuration to create a herring bone pattern (See Diagram D). Secure the wrap on the upper thigh with two clips. Do not finish the clips on the inside of the thigh as they could cut the opposite thigh or just pop off.
- Secure the wrap with one 3" elastic tape strip while the athlete contracts his/her thigh muscles (See Diagram D).

QUADRICEPS SUPPORT (OPTION)

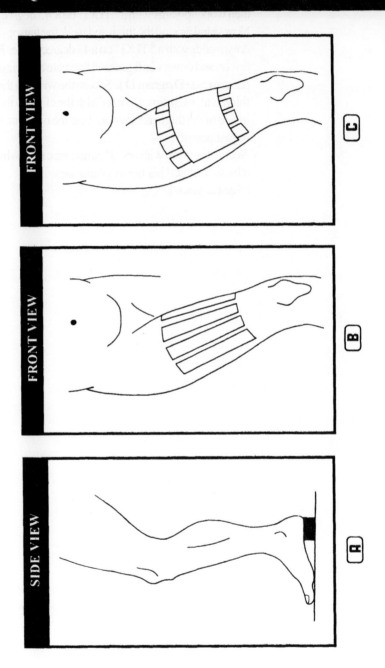

80

QUADRICEPS SUPPORT (OPTION)

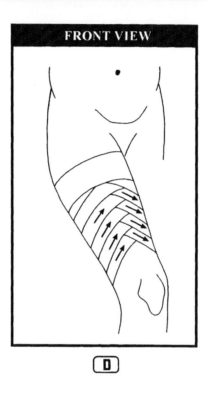

FRONT VIEW

D

HAMSTRING SUPPORT

PURPOSE: - To provide compression to a strain or a contusion in the acute stage.

SUPPLIES: - tuf-skin spray
- underwrap
- pressure pad
- 1 1/2" and 2" white adhesive tape
- 6" tensor bandage
- 3" elastic tape

IMPORTANT TEACHING POINTS:
SKIN PREPARATION
AND
BODY POSITIONING
- The athlete should be standing.
- Shave the hair from the back of the thigh.
- Spray the thigh with tuf-skin.
- Apply a pressure pad over the area of injury.

ANCHORS - Secure one 2" white adhesive tape strip on the outside of the injured area and one 2" white adhesive tape strip on the inside of the injured area (See Diagram A).

SUPPORT TECHNIQUE - Start the first compression strip just below the area of injury on the inner back of the thigh, travelling upwards on a 45 degree angle (See Diagram B). The next support strip starts on the outside anchor of the back of the thigh. From here the strip travels upwards to the inside of the thigh on a 45 degree angle.
- Repeat the above strips while overlapping by half the width of the tape until the area is fully covered (See Diagram C). The tape strips do not go completely around the thigh (See Diagram D). Cover the support with underwrap. This decreases the possibilty of the wrap moving or sliding during activity.

82

CLOSURES

- Close the entire tape job with a 6" tensor bandage.
- Have the athlete contract the muscle.
- Start to apply the tensor below the injury and then work upwards with a " TUG " on a 45 degree angle. Now spiral around the thigh and work the tensor downwards with a " TUG " on a 45 degree angle as well.
- Repeat this up and down configuration to create a herring bone pattern (See Diagram E).
- Secure the wrap with three clips. Do not finish the clips on the inside of the leg as they could rub and cut the opposite leg or just pop off. Secure the wrap with one 3" elastic tape strip (See Diagram E).

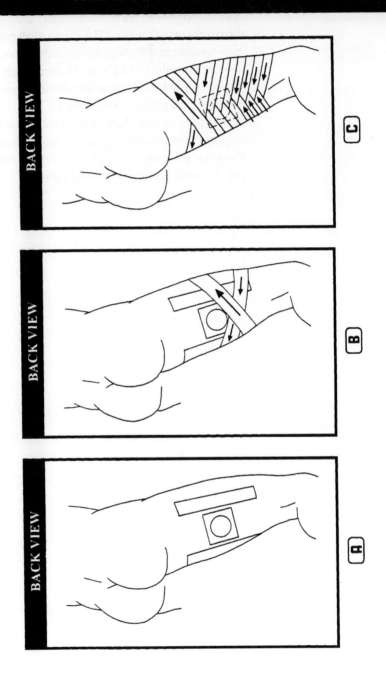

HAMSTRING SUPPORT

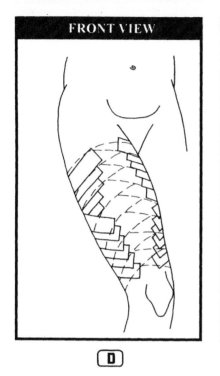

FRONT VIEW

D

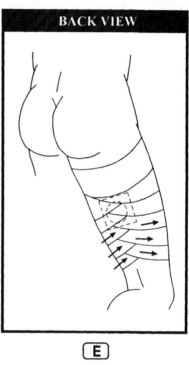

BACK VIEW

E

85

HIP FLEXOR-GROIN WRAP

PURPOSE: - To provide support for a hip flexor and/or adductor strain.

SUPPLIES: - underwrap
- 6" double length tensor, or two 6" regular tensor bandages
- 2" or 3" white adhesive tape
- tuf-skin spray
- 3" elastic tape

IMPORTANT TEACHING POINTS:
SKIN PREPARATION
AND
BODY POSITIONING

- Spray the upper thigh with tuf-skin. Underwrap the thigh, this will help keep the wrap from slipping.
- Position the athlete by placing a 1 1/2" roll of adhesive tape under the heel. The knee should be bent at an angle of 10-15 degrees while bending slightly forward with the hip flexed (See Diagram A).
- Rotate the lower leg inward slightly. Have the toes pointing in.

SUPPORT TECHNIQUE

- Secure the tensor bandage mid-thigh while wrapping towards the inner thigh (See Diagram B) and then spiral around the thigh three times (See Diagram C). Now proceed upwards with a quick tug on the tensor bandage (See Diagram C).
- Carry the tensor bandage around the back, level with the top of the hip bone.
- Travel downwards (See Diagram E) and around the thigh.

CLOSURES

- Repeat this " figure 8 " procedure at least 3 times. Secure the tensor bandage on the upper thigh with three 2" white adhesive tape strips over the tensor clips (See Diagram F). Do not apply these strips too tightly. To accomplish this, have the athlete contract his/her thigh muscles prior to applying the tape.
- When finished, the support technique should help spring the thigh upwards. It will also limit how far the athlete can abduct and externally rotate his/ her thigh.

CLOSURE OPTION

- Cover the entire procedure with one 3" elastic tape " figure 8 ", starting and finishing at the thigh. Secure the elastic tape with two 2" white adhesive tape strips. Be sure to have the athlete contract the thigh muscles before securing the white adhesive tape.

HIP FLEXOR-GROIN WRAP

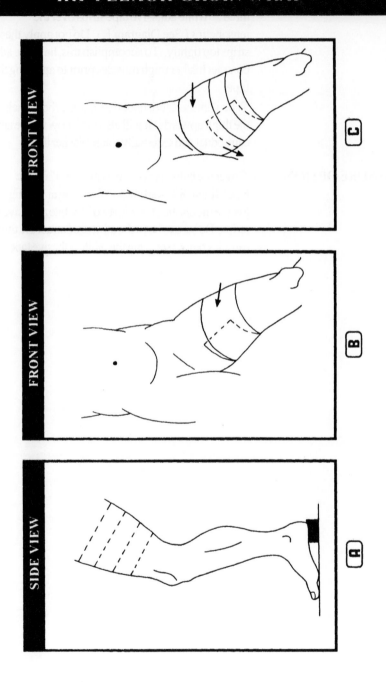

FRONT VIEW

C

FRONT VIEW

B

SIDE VIEW

A

HIP FLEXOR-GROIN WRAP

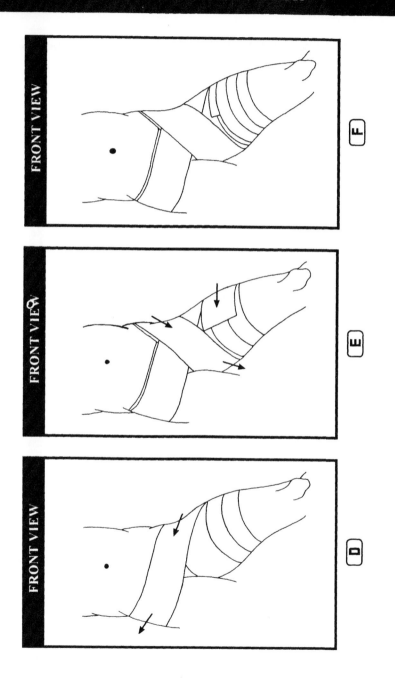

FRONT VIEW

F

FRONT VIEW

E

FRONT VIEW

D

CHAPTER FIVE

SHOULDER-AC JOINT PROTECTION

SHOULDER-SPICA WRAP

SHOULDER-PREVENT ANTERIOR DISLOCATION

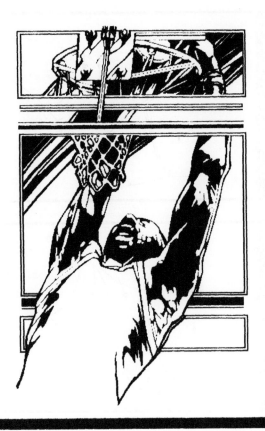

SHOULDER-AC JOINT PROTECTION

PURPOSE: - To provide support and protection to an acromio
    clavicular (AC) joint.

SUPPLIES: - tuf-skin spray
    - felt or adhesive foam (1/2" thick) (SanSplint is optional)
    - 3" elastic tape
    - heel & lace pads
    - 2" elastic tape
    - 1 1/2" white adhesive tape
    - band-aids (2 knuckle)
    - skin lubricant

IMPORTANT TEACHING POINTS:
SKIN PREPARATION
AND
BODY POSITIONING - Shave the area around the chest and arm prior
    to taping.
    - Spray the arm and chest with tuf-skin.
    - Cover the nipples with heel and lace pads or with a
    band-aid and some skin lubricant.
    - The arm should be supported on a table.
    - Apply a donut pad over the AC joint (See diagram A).
    A hard shell placed over the donut will provide good
    protection.

ANCHORS - Apply a 3" elastic tape anchor from the nipple,
    passing upwards over the clavicle and then
    down to the shoulder blade (See Diagram A).
    - Apply a 3" elastic tape anchor over the biceps muscle
    (mid-biceps). Have the athlete tighten the muscle
    before securing the tape.
    - Apply a 3" elastic tape anchor around the chest. Be
    sure to have the athlete inhale before securing the tape
    (See Diagram A).

91

SUPPORT TECHNIQUE- Use 1 1/2" white adhesive tape to create the following support strips. The first support strip should begin on the outer part of the back of the arm then work upwards to end on the front of the chest.
- The next strip should begin on the front of the arm while crossing over the first support strip to end on the shoulder blade. This will create an " X " pattern over the AC joint.
- Repeat the above " X " pattern until the AC joint is covered (See Diagram B).
- Usually three to four strips in each direction is adequate.

CLOSURES
- Close the biceps with two 2" elastic tape strips. Be sure to have the athlete flex the arm before closing the strips.
- Close the area above the nipple by using 2" elastic tape strips passing upwards from the nipple and finishing on the shoulder blade anchor. Repeat three or four times and overlap each strip by half the width of the tape (See Diagram C).
- Apply three 1 1/2" white adhesive tape strip closures which start at the nipple and go horizontally around the chest to finish at the shoulder blade. Overlap each strip by half the width of the tape (See Diagram C).
- Finish the closure by using 3" elastic tape around the chest. Have the athlete inhale before securing the tape closure (See Diagram D).
- Secure the end of the tape with three 1 1/2" white adhesive tape strips (See Diagram D).
- A tight-fitting shirt should be worn by the athlete to keep this support technique in place.

SHOULDER-AC JOINT PROTECTION

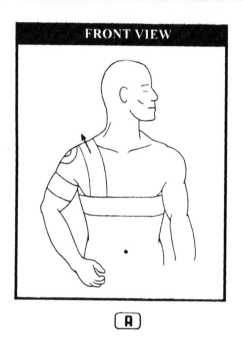

A

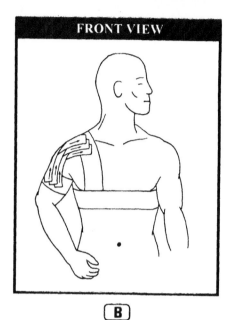

B

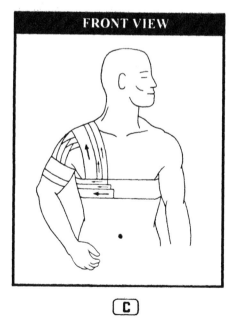

C

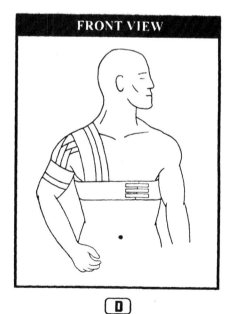

D

SHOULDER-SPICA WRAP

PURPOSE: - To help prevent abduction and external rotation of the shoulder.

SUPPLIES: - tuf-skin spray   - 6" double length tensor bandage
           - 2" elastic tape   - band-aid

IMPORTANT TEACHING POINTS:
SKIN PREPARATION
AND
BODY POSITIONING
- Position the athlete with their arm internally rotated, as if their hand were in their back pocket (See Diagram A).
- Cover the nipple with skin lube and a band-aid. Have the athlete tighten upper arm muscles during the wrap procedure.
- Spray the arm and chest lightly with tuf-skin.

SUPPORT TECHNIQUE
AND CLOSURE
- Begin the wrap by securing it around the biceps (See Diagram B). The wrap must start on the outside of the arm, wrap inwards under the arm pit then carry outwards and around the arm again. The wrap should now continue across the chest, under the opposite arm and then traverse upwards around the affected shoulder again (See Diagram C).
- Repeat this procedure (See Diagram D) then clip the tensor at the arm (See Diagram E).
- Position the clips on the biceps and then cover with two 2" elastic tape strips (See Diagram F). Make sure to contract biceps muscles prior to applying the closures.
- Do not finish the tensor wrap so that the clips are next to the chest. The clips could come undone or injure the skin (See Diagram E).

94

SHOULDER-SPICA WRAP

FRONT VIEW

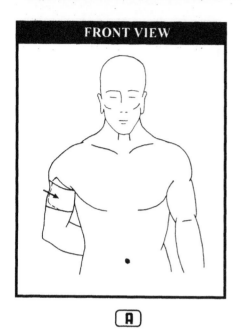

A

FRONT VIEW

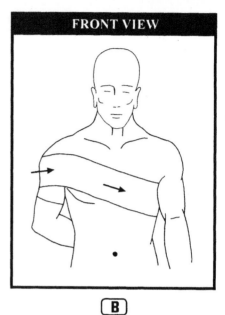

B

FRONT VIEW

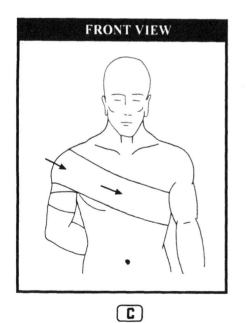

C

BACK VIEW

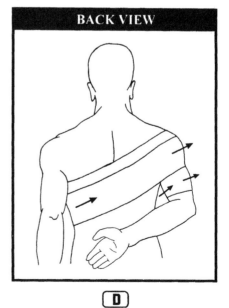

D

SHOULDER-SPICA WRAP

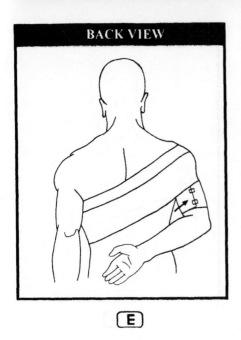

E

BACK VIEW

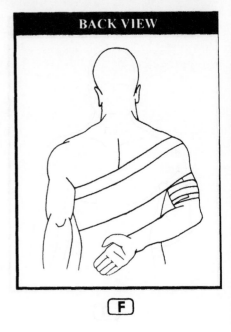

F

96

SHOULDER-PREVENT ANT. DISLOCATION

PURPOSE: - To provide support for the Gleno- Humeral joint by limiting abduction and external rotation.

SUPPLIES: - tuf-skin spray
- 3" elastic tape
- 1 1/2" white adhesive tape

IMPORTANT TEACHING POINTS:
SKIN PREPARATION
    AND
BODY POSITIONING - The arm and chest should first be shaved and then sprayed with tuf-skin.
- The athlete should be positioned such that his/ her arm is in a resting position with the hand near the belly button.

ANCHORS - Secure one 3" elastic tape anchor around the biceps while having the athlete contract the muscle (See Diagram A).
- Secure one 3" elastic tape anchor around the chest. The athlete must inhale first before securing the tape (See Diagram A).

SUPPORT TECHNIQUE- Begin a 3" elastic tape support strip mid-chest then travel horizontally around the chest and the affected arm to finish near the beginning of the strip (See Diagram B). Pinch the tape together between the arm and the chest to create a checkrein.

97

CLOSURES

- Close the support technique with 3" elastic tape starting on the outside of the arm (See Diagram C). Now travel horizontally across the chest, behind the back and around the affected arm again. Finish this 3" elastic tape strip just near the side of the chest wall (See Diagram C).
- Pinch the elastic tape together again between the arm and chest. Wrap several 1 1/2" white adhesive tape strips around the checkrein that has been established between the arm and the chest (See Diagram C).

SHOULDER-PREVENT ANT. DISLOCATION

FRONT VIEW

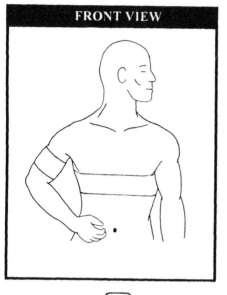

A

FRONT VIEW

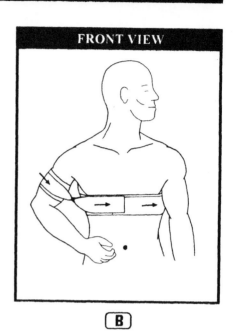

B

FRONT VIEW

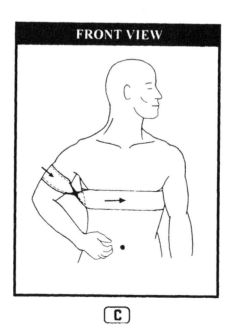

C

CHAPTER SIX

ELBOW-HYPEREXTENSION SUPPORT

WRIST-HYPEREXTENSION SUPPORT

THUMB-HYPEREXTENSION SUPPORT

THUMB HYPEREXTENSION (CHECKREIN)

FINGER (BUDDY TAPING)

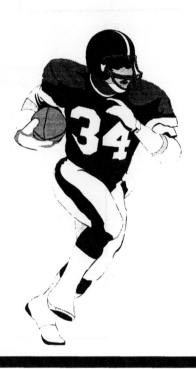

ELBOW-HYPEREXTENSION SUPPORT

PURPOSE: - To prevent the elbow from hyperextention.

SUPPLIES: - tuf-skin spray
- 1 1/2" white adhesive tape
- 2" and 3" elastic tape
- skin lubricant

IMPORTANT TEACHING POINTS:
SKIN PREPARATION
AND
BODY POSITIONING

- Shave the upper and lower arm.
- Spray the upper and lower arm with tuf-skin.
- Position the elbow in a slightly bent position.

ANCHORS

- Apply two 2" elastic tape anchors around the mid-forearm. Overlap each strip by half the width of the tape. Make sure the athlete makes a fist and contracts forearm musculature (See Diagram A).
- Apply two 3" elastic tape anchors around the biceps muscle. The first anchor is placed around the mid-biceps and the second anchor is placed above the belly of the biceps. Overlap each piece by half the width of the tape. Have the athlete contract the biceps before securing the anchors (See Diagram A). This can be done by resisting flexion at the elbow with the opposite hand.

CHECKREIN
FORMATION

- Once the painfree angle of the elbow has been established, measure the distance from the top of one anchor to the bottom of the other by using the white adhesive tape. Lay this strip on a table and add four to six more to it to create a fan shaped checkrein. The amount of added strips will depend on the size of the arm. Secure a 1 1/2" white adhesive tape piece around the center of the checkrein (See Diagram B).
- Position the pre-formed checkrein (See Diagram C), then secure the forearm first with two 2" elastic tape strips (See Diagram D).
- Overlap each piece by half the width of the tape.
- Now secure the checkrein on the biceps, again with two 2" elastic tape strips, each overlapped by half the width of the tape.

CLOSURES

- Apply one 3" elastic tape piece over the mid-biceps. Close the area beyond the biceps muscle with one 2" adhesive tape strip. Have the athlete contract the biceps before applying both closures (See Diagram D).

OPTION

- An additional checkrein can be made and applied to the medial aspect of the arm to protect the medial collateral ligaments.

ELBOW-HYPEREXTENSION SUPPORT

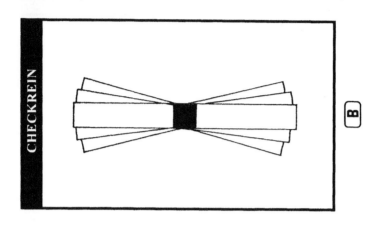

CHECKREIN

B

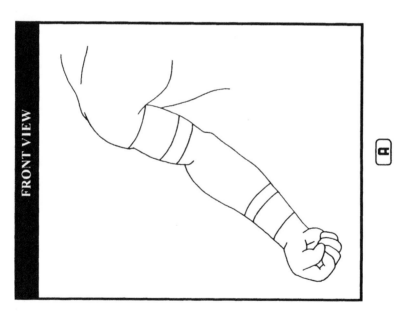

FRONT VIEW

A

ELBOW-HYPEREXTENSION SUPPORT

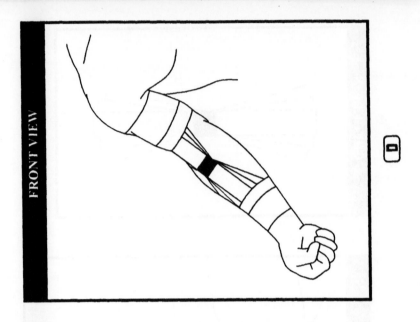

FRONT VIEW

D

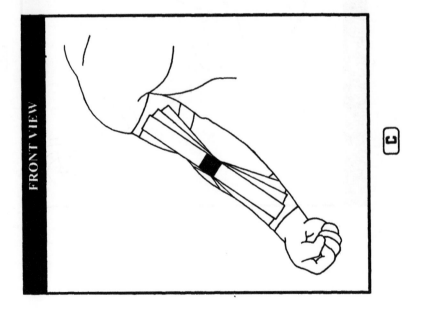

FRONT VIEW

C

WRIST-HYPEREXTENSION SUPPORT

PURPOSE: - To prevent excessive wrist extension. (This same technique
               can be used to prevent hyper flexion).

SUPPLIES: - tuf-skin spray
              - underwrap
              - 1" or 1 1/2" white adhesive tape
              - 1/2" white adhesive tape

IMPORTANT TEACHING POINTS:
SKIN PREPARATION
AND
BODY POSITIONING
- Shave the forearm to be taped.
- Spray the forearm and hand with tuf-skin.
  Apply underwrap only at the crease of the wrist. This
  will prevent friction and blisters.
- Have the athlete hold the wrist in a straight position
  (neutral) with the fingers spread apart.
- Place the athlete's fingers against your stomach to
  prevent any movement of the wrist during the taping
  procedure.

ANCHORS
- Use 1 1/2" white adhesive tape to create three
  wrist anchors. The first wrist anchor starts at the crease
  in the wrist. The other two anchors continue up the
  forearm from here and are overlapped by half the width
  of the tape. Do not pass the muscle belly of the
  forearm.
- The fourth anchor starts and finishes on the back
  of the hand (See Diagram A). Make sure the fingers
  are spread apart.
- Be sure to fold the white adhesive tape when passing
  over the web of the thumb.
- Do not cover the knuckles of the fingers as the
  athlete should be able to make a fist.

- The fifth anchor starts at the wrist on a slight angle. This piece travels down the inside of the wrist, over the back of the hand, down the palm and finishes at the base of the thumb (See Diagrams B & C). Be sure to fold the edges of the tape over when crossing the web of the thumb.
- Apply one last anchor (sixth) at the base of the thumb, starting on the back of the hand and finishing in the palm (See Diagram D).

CHECKREIN SUPPORT

- Measure the required length of the checkrein by measuring from one anchor to the other with 1" or 1 1/2" white adhesive tape.
- Once the length has been established, form an " X " on top of the piece of 1" or 1 1/2" white adhesive tape (See Diagram E).

CLOSURES

- Begin the closure of the tape job by repeating the fourth anchor. This will be called closure number one (C1) (See Diagram G).
- Now take the checkrein and pull the wrist into slight flexion while securing the checkrein onto the forearm (See Diagram F). If too long, fold it back.
- Secure the forearm with three overlapping closure strips of 1 1/2" white adhesive tape (C2, C3, C4) (See Diagram G).
- Now check the function of the wrist.

OPTION

- For extra support secure one or two 1/2" white adhesive tape strips over the crease in the wrist (See Diagram H).

106

WRIST-HYPEREXTENSION SUPPORT

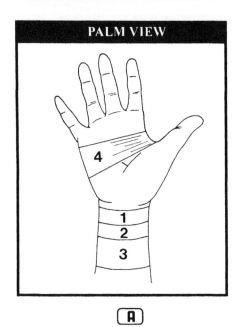

PALM VIEW

A

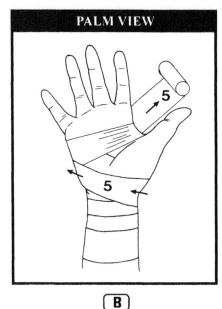

PALM VIEW

B

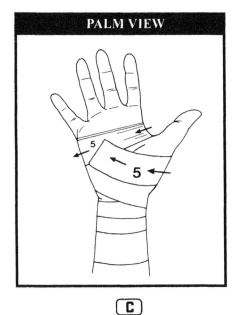

PALM VIEW

C

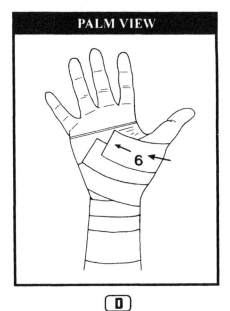

PALM VIEW

D

WRIST-HYPEREXTENSION SUPPORT

PALM VIEW

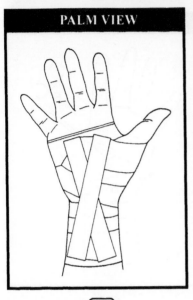

E

SIDE VIEW

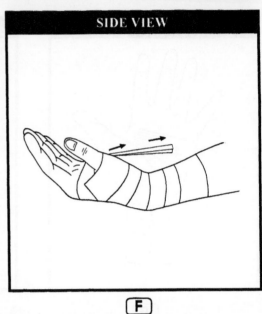

F

PALM VIEW

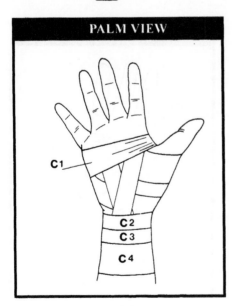

C1

C2
C3

C4

G

BACK VIEW

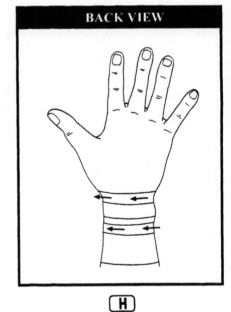

H

THUMB-HYPEREXTENSION SUPPORT

PURPOSE: - To prevent hyperextension of the thumb.

SUPPLIES: - tuf-skin spray
- 1 1/2" white adhesive tape

IMPORTANT TEACHING POINTS:
SKIN PREPARATION
    AND
BODY POSITIONING - The hand is supported on the therapist's chest or stomach.
- The thumb should be placed in a functional position and in its pain free range (See Diagram A).
- Spray the entire hand & thumb with tuf-skin.

ANCHORS - Using 1 1/2" white adhesive tape, the first anchor should start on the front of the wrist (See Diagram B), wrap around the back of the hand and over the web of the thumb (See Diagram C). As the tape passes over the web of the thumb, pinch the edges to prevent the tape from cutting the skin.
- Continue the anchor down the palm and around the back of the wrist to finish on the front of the wrist (See Diagram C).
- This strip can be repeated for more stability and support (optional).

HOOD FORMATION
    &
SUPPORT TECHNIQUE - Using 1 1/2" white adhesive tape strips, start the hood on the back of the anchor at the base of the thumb, wrap around and attach onto the front of the anchor (See Diagram D).
- Repeat these strips by continuing up the thumb and overlapping by half the width of the tape each time (See Diagram E).

- The number of hoods required will depend on the length of the thumb.
- Make sure the proximal joint is covered.
- Pinch the edges of the last hood piece together in order to help prevent hyperextension. The last hood piece should not interfere with the bending of the tip of the thumb.
- The degree of hyperextension restriction will depend upon the positioning of the thumb.

CLOSURES

- To close, re-apply the original hand anchor to secure the hood pieces (See Diagram F).

OPTION
HYPERABDUCTION SUPPORT

"FIGURE 8"

- To prevent the thumb from opening up into abduction, apply two " figure 8 " strips travelling in the same direction (See Diagrams G & H). The two strips should begin on the back of the hand, loop around the base of the thumb and end in the palm. The " X's " should cross over the MTP joint. These strips should be applied before the closures.
- Do not apply the tape too tight as it is easy to cut off circulation.

THUMB-HYPEREXTENSION SUPPORT

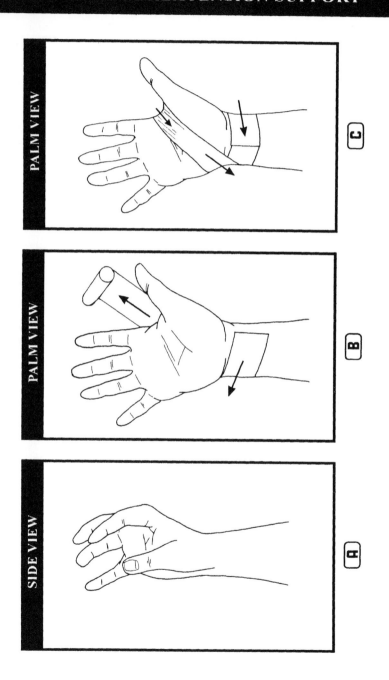

PALM VIEW

C

PALM VIEW

B

SIDE VIEW

A

THUMB-HYPEREXTENSION SUPPORT

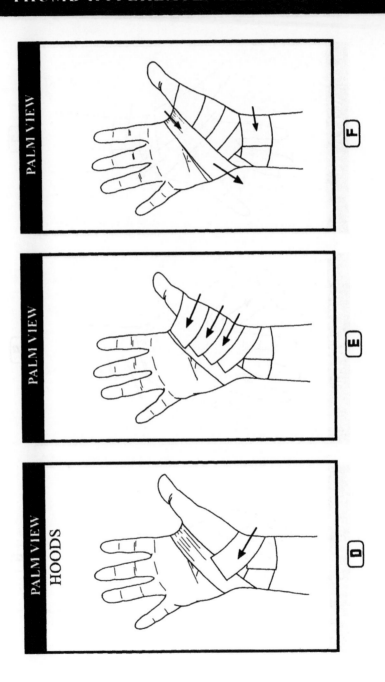

112

THUMB-HYPEREXTENSION SUPPORT

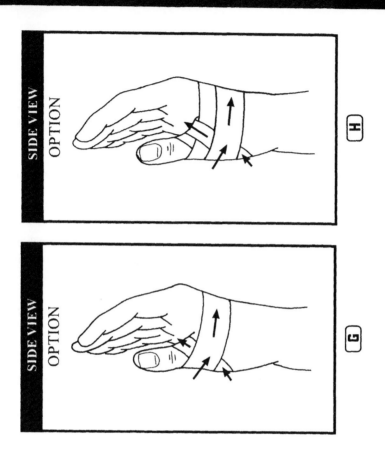

SIDE VIEW OPTION H

SIDE VIEW OPTION G

THUMB HYPEREXTENSION (CHECKREIN)

PURPOSE: - To prevent hyperextension of the thumb.

SUPPLIES: - tuf-skin spray
- 1" white adhesive tape

IMPORTANT TEACHING POINTS:
SKIN PREPARATION
    AND
BODY POSITIONING - Position the thumb in a functional pain-free range of extension (See Diagram A).
- Spray the thumb and index finger with tuf-skin.

ANCHORS - Using 1" white adhesive tape, apply one anchor to the first digit of the thumb and one anchor to the first digit of the index finger (See Diagram A).

SUPPORT TECHNIQUE - Secure the two digits together with a 1" white adhesive tape loop, thus joining the two fingers together. Pinch the tape together between the fingers to create a checkrein (See Diagram B).
- Apply a final 1" tape closure over the tape that has been pinched together (See Diagram B).
- Be sure that the index finger joints and the thumb joints can flex properly.
- Check the function of the support technique.

114

THUMB HYPEREXTENSION (CHECKREIN)

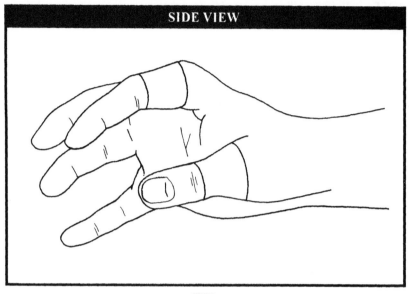

SIDE VIEW

A

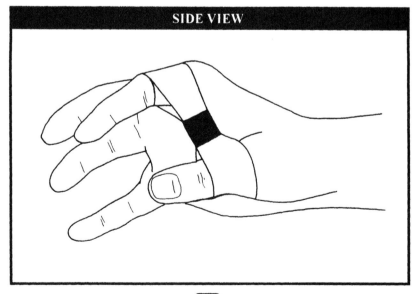

SIDE VIEW

B

115

FINGER (BUDDY TAPING)

PURPOSE: - To immobilize an injured finger joint or
as a measure to prevent finger injury.

SUPPLIES: - tuf-skin spray
- 3" x 3" gauze pads
- 1 1/2" and 1" white adhesive tape

IMPORTANT TEACHING POINTS:
SKIN PREPARATION
SUPPORT TECHNIQUE

- Spray the two fingers with tuf-skin.
- Cut gauze, felt or foam to fit between the injured and non-injured " support " finger.
- Preference for buddy taping involves pairing fingers # 1, # 2 and # 3, # 4 by taping above and below the injured joint (See Diagram A).
- Finish by tearing the tape on the back of the hand to prevent the tape from unwinding (See Diagram A).

FINGER (BUDDY TAPING)

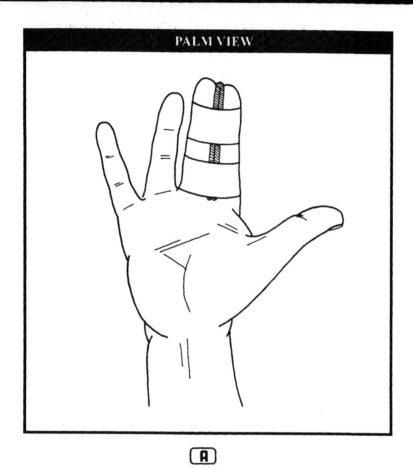

PALM VIEW

A

CHAPTER SEVEN

GLOSSARY

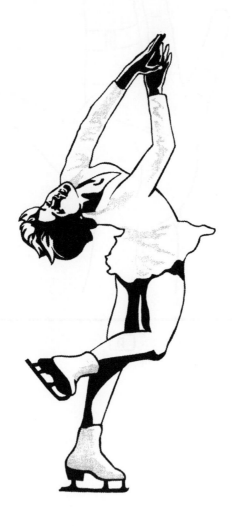

GLOSSARY

Abduction: The lateral movement of a limb away from the median plane of the body.

Acute: Immediate injury onset associated with inflammation.

Adduction: The movement of a body segment toward the median anatomical line of a nearby segment.

Anterior: The front of the body or a body part.

Articulation: A joint between bones.

Avulsion: A forcible tearing away of a part or structure (i.e., a ligament from a bone).

Axilla: Arm pit.

Bursa: A fluid-filled sac or sac-like cavity that allows a muscle or tendon to slide over bone thereby reducing friction.

Checkrein: Several strips of tape that run between upper and lower anchors. It is often shaped like an hour glass.

Chronic Injury :   an injury showing little change or slow improvement. The opposite of acute.

Dislocation: The displacement of one or more bones, a joint, or any organ from it's original position.

Distal: Farthest from a center, from the midline, or from the trunk. Farthest from a point of reference (opposite of proximal).

Dorsal: Upper surface (i.e., top of hand/ foot)

Dorsiflexion:	Moving the toe or foot, finger or wrist, toward the dorsal aspect of a nearby body segment.
Dorsum:	The back of a body part.
Edema:	Swelling as a result of the collection of fluid in the connective tissue.
Effusion:	Escape of the fluid into a cavity (such as within a joint capsule).
Epiphysis:	A growth plate.
Eversion:	Moving the soles of the feet so that they are facing away from each other.
Extension:	Moving a body segment toward a straight line position.
Fascia:	Fibrous membrane that covers, supports, and separates muscles.
Fascitis:	Inflammation of fascia.
Flexion:	Moving a body segment away from a straight line position.
Forefoot:	The area of the foot before the toes (arch area).
Heel & Lace Pads:	A 3" X 3" closed cell foam pad, 2 - 3 mm thick, designed to protect the skin.
Hematoma:	A bruise, consisting of a collection of blood that is usually clotted.
Hemorrhage:	Escaping of blood through ruptured walls of blood vessels.
Hyper:	Prefix meaning too much (i.e., hyperextension).

Hyper-
Extension: Beyond the normal extension.

Hyperflexion: In excess of normal flexion.

Hypo-:   Prefix signifying a lack of or deficiency; also a position below, under or beneath.

Inferior: Towards the bottom of the body or body part.

Insertion: Muscle attachment to a bone that moves.

Inversion: Moving the feet so that the soles face each other.

itis: A suffix, an inflammation of something (i.e., tendonitis)

Joint Capsule: (articular capsule or synovial capsule) A saclike, fibrous membrane that surrounds a joint, often including or interwoven with ligaments.

Joint
Subluxation: Partial displacement of the articular surfaces between two or more bones.

Lateral: Away from the midline of the body. Pertains to the side (in relationship of position from the midline of the body).

Ligament: A band of flexible, tough, dense white fibrous connective tissue connecting the articular ends of the bones and sometimes enveloping them in a capsule.

Malleolus: A rounded bony protuberance on each side of the ankle joint.

Medial: Toward the midline of the body.

Medium
Density Foam: Similar to that found in hockey helmets

Muscle:	A tissue composed of contractile fibers or cells. A contractile organ composed of muscle tissue.
Myositis Ossificans:	Inflammation of muscle, with the formation of bone tissue in it.
Neutral:	Indifferent, or neither extreme.
Non Tearing Tape:	Tape that must be cut with scissors - will not tear.
Origin:	The fixed end or attachment of a muscle, ligament etc...
Palmar:	Pertaining to the palm of the hand.
Phalanges:	Bones of the fingers and toes.
Plantar:	Ventral aspect of the foot (sole of the foot).
Plantar Flexion:	Moving the toe or foot toward the plantar aspect of a nearby body part. (i.e., Pointing the toe and foot).
Popliteal Space:	The area behind the knee joint.
Posterior:	The back of the body or a body part.
Prone:	Face- down, horizontal position of the body.
Prophylactic:	Any agent or regimen that contributes to the prevention of an injury or disease.
Proximal:	An area closest to the point of attachment, origin, or point of reference.
Separation:	Injury to a general non- movable joint (i.e., an AC Joint separation).

Spica: Continuous strips of tape or a tensor that wrap around a joint forming a " figure 8 ".

Sprain: An overstress of a joint, producing a stretching or tearing of the ligaments and capsule.

Strain: Excessive stretching or overuse of a part, such as a tendon or a muscle.

Superior: Towards the top of the body or body part.

Splay: To spread apart or move outward.

Supine: Lying on the back. facing upwards, opposed to prone.

Tendon: A band of dense fibrous tissue forming the termination of a muscle and attaching the latter to a bone.

Tuff-skin: A sticky skin adherent spray.

Turf-Toe: A toe injury resulting from the big toe being forced against the tip of the shoe. This results in excessive hyper extension of the MP joint.

Underwrap: A thin, tearable wrap used as a protective barrier against the skin. It comes by the roll and is also know as under wrap or pre-wrap.

Valgus: Position of a body part that is bent outward away from the midline of the body.

Varus: Position of a body part that is bent inward toward the midline of the body.

Ventral: Bottom surface (opposite of dorsal); near, on, or toward the belly; in human, anterior.

ABOUT THE AUTHOR

Robert Kennedy is the President of FITNESS TECH PRODUCTS INC., a growing company that is involved in the designing, manufacturing, and marketing of fitness equipment worldwide. In 1984, he received his honours degree in Physical Education from the University of Ottawa. Over the past several years, he has been involved in the sports medicine field as a sports therapist. During this time, he has worked at the University of Ottawa Sports Medicine Clinic with a number of different inter-collegiate teams. In addition, he has been actively involved with several national, professional, and amateur athletic teams.

NOTES

NOTES

NOTES

NOTES

NOTES

NOTES

NOTES

Printed and bound by CPI Group (UK) Ltd, Croydon, CR0 4YY

08/06/2025

01896874-0003